ORTHOPEDICS

The REGENTS/PRENTICE HALL
MEDICAL ASSISTANT KIT

ORTHOPEDICS

Third Edition

REGENTS/PRENTICE HALL, Englewood Cliffs, New Jersey 07632

Library of Congress Cataloging in Publication Data
Orthopedics. — 3rd. ed.
p. cm. — (The Regents/Prentice Hall medical assistant kit)
Includes index.
ISBN 0-13-156845-0
[DNLM: 1. Orthopedics. WE 168 0726275]
rd731.0787 1992
617.3—DC20
DNLM/DLC
for Library of Congress 92-48840
CIP

A Division of Simon & Schuster
Englewood Cliffs, NJ 07632

Notice
The information and procedures described in the REGENTS/PRENTICE HALL MEDICAL ASSISTANT KIT are based on consultation with practitioners and instructors and are to be used as part of a formal course taught by a qualified Medical Assistant instructor. To the best of the publisher's knowledge, this information reflects currently accepted practices; however, it cannot be considered absolute recommendations. For individual application, the policies and procedures of the institution or agency where the Medical Assistant is employed must be reviewed and followed. The authors of these materials and their supplements disclaim responsiblity for any adverse effects resulting directly or indirectly from the suggested procedures and theory, from any undetected errors, or from the reader's misunderstanding of the materials. It is the reader's responsiblity to stay informed of any new changes or recommendations made by his or her employing health care institution or agency.

Printed in the United States of America

10 9 8 7 6 5 4 3 2 1

ISBN 0-13-156845-0

Prentice-Hall International (UK) Limited, *London*
Prentice-Hall of Australia, Pty Limited, *Sydney*
Prentice-Hall Canada, Inc., *Toronto*
Prentice-Hall Hispanoamericana, S.A., *Mexico*
Prentice-Hall of India Private Limited, *New Delhi*
Prentice-Hall of Japan, Inc., *Tokyo*
Simon & Shuster Asia Pte. Ltd., *Singapore*
Editora Prentice-Hall do Brasil, Ltda., *Rio de Janeiro*

Contents

Preface

The REGENTS/PRENTICE HALL MEDICAL ASSISTANT KIT is the only textbook series written for students of Medical Assisting, which integrates the study of anatomy and physiology with diagnosis and treatment of disease. Our goal in this revision was to update and improve the series.

To achieve this goal, we solicited the advice of long-time users of the kit. Their comments resulted in many basic changes including simplification of concepts and procedures; addition of up-to-date information; an emphasis on quality control in all aspects of the physician's office laboratory; and enhanced study aids.

SIMPLIFICATION AND UP-TO-DATE INFORMATION

- All the books are infection-control–conscious throughout, reflecting the latest OSHA regulations.
- Anatomy and physiology titles have been simplified to reflect the very practical approach taken by many instructors.
- Diagnoses and treatments of disease have been up-dated for each body system.
- A thoroughly revised *Bio-Organization* launches the anatomy and physiology series with a simplified introduction to the structure and function of the body and a solid foundation for the study of human disease.
- *Laboratory Processes for Medical Assisting* is revised with more than 60% new material including performance-based procedure checklists for easy instructor evaluation, and the latest requirements of the Clinical Laboratory Improvement Act (CLIA).
- *Clinical Processes for Medical Assisting* now emphasizes only clinical procedures in the POL, leaving administrative issues to other more specific courses.

EMPHASIS ON QUALITY CONTROL

As the federal, state and local regulations become more specific, it is clear that the physician's major challenge is to provide not only the highest level of quality care and treatment for the patient, but also to document his or her commitment to that quality for the interest of government. It most often falls on the shoulders of the medical assistant to execute and police the quality control procedures within the office. The new laboratory books emphasize this need for quality control documentation.

The popular "Sources of Error" within the laboratory and clinical procedures checklists have been scrutinized and amplified.

ENHANCED STUDY AIDS

- Knowledge Objectives are grouped by chapter and by section.
- Pronunciations of medical terms are provided the first time a word is used. New terms appear in bold type and are defined in the extensive updated glossary.
- STOP AND REVIEW sections reflect Knowledge Objectives by section or by chapter.
- Over 60 new or revised illustrations and tables complement the text.
- All illustrations and tables are now precisely referenced in the text.
- Contemporary "sidebars" add spice and topical information to entice the student.
- Redesigned books emphasize organization and easy reading.
- Two new simplified four-color inserts are: A blood cell chart showing normal and abnormal blood cells; and 12 pages of body systems illustrations to accompany the *Bio-Organization* introduction.
- *Clinical Processes for Medical Assisting* includes the same type procedure checklist as *Laboratory Processes for Medical Assisting* for easy instructor evaluation.

PREVIOUS BENEFITS RETAINED

The same strengths and benefits which instructors valued in the past have been retained or expanded:

- The flexible modular format can adjust to various program lengths or different orders of coverage for laboratory, clinical, and anatomy and physiology topics.
- The kit is written in a style specifically appropriate to the medical assisting student.
- The text/workbook style aids student learning. The material remains in small, manageable segments.
- The kit takes an integrated approach to structure, function, and disease of the human body.
- Each body system or medical specialty is followed by its clinical counterpoint of disease, diagnosis and treatment.
- A thorough review of disorders and diseases is classified by type in *Bio-Organization*, and by system through the subsequent anatomy and physiology 10-book series.
- The kit features an emphasis on quality control in *Laboratory Processes for Medical Assisting* and *Clinical Processes for Medical Assisting*.
- No prior knowledge of biology or chemistry is assumed.

ACKNOWLEDGMENTS

The revision of the Medical Assistant Kit represents a cooperative effort among many people. Foremost is Debra Grieneisen, M.T., C.M.A., who served as advisor for the series and in-depth reviser for *Laboratory Process for Medical Assisting*. Debra has taught medical assisting at Harrisburg Area Community College and Central Pennsylvania Business School, and it is her commitment to perfection that guided this work.

Several medical writers contributed to these books. Thank you to:

Karen Garloff, R.N.
Bruce Goldfarb
Steve Hulse
Ann Moy
Joy Nixon, R.N.

Cindy Jennings of BMR lead the editorial efforts to manage this revision. Helping her were Nancy Priff and Rick Stull, as well as Jacqueline Flynn and Greg Flynn.

We particularly want to thank the reviewers whose advice, recommendations and collective knowledge helped form these books. Their concern for the subject matter, its accuracy, and primarily their students' best interest are reflected here. One thing they all agreed upon is the importance of accurate, clear illustrations which are integrated and referenced throughout the text. Our reviewers were:

Joanne Bakel
Milton S. Hershey Medical Center
Hershey, PA

Linda Barrer
Lansdale Business School
Lansdale, PA

Judy Bettinger
Private Medical Practice
Camp Hill, PA

C. Michael Cronin
California College of Health Sciences
National City, CA

Martha Faison
Private Medical Practice
Camp Hill, PA

Irene Figliolina
Berdan Institute
Totowa, NJ

Kathleen Hess
Antonelli Medical & Professional Institute
Pottstown, PA

Carol Kish
Harrisburg Hospital
Harrisburg, PA

Peter Kish
Harrisburg Area Community College
Harrisburg, PA

Tibby Loveman
Gadsden Business College
Gadsden, AL

Scott McKenzie
Commonwealth College
Virginia Beach, VA

Pat Morelli
Medical Careers Training Center
Ft. Collins, CO

Rhonda O'Grady
The Laboratory Arts Institute
Scarborough, Ontario

Sheila Ritchey
Harrisburg Hospital
Harrisburg, PA

Sandy Rishell
Private Medical Practice
Harrisburg, PA

Janet Sesser
The Bryman School
Phoenix, AZ

Shirley Seekford
Antonelli Medical &
Professional Institute
Pottstown, PA

Robert Sheperd Kee
Business College
Norfolk, VA

Laura Silva
The Sawyer School
Pawtucket, RI

Pamela Smith
Private Medical Practice
Harrisburg, PA

Bruce Sundrud
Harrisburg Area Community
College
Harrisburg, PA

Ann Sugarman
Berdan Institute
Totowa, NJ

Dan Tallman
Northern State University
Aberdeen, SD

Jackie Trentacosta
Galen College
Fresno, CA

Fred Ann Tull
Southern Technical College
Little Rick, AR

Deborah Wood
Concorde Career Institute
Lauderdale Lakes, FL

And finally, those who gave detailed feedback on our questionnaires helped configure the kit in its present form:

Theresa Bowser
Southern Ohio College
Columbus, OH

Elaine Chamberlin
Pontiac Business Institute
Oxford, MI

Thelma Clavon
Rutledge College
Columbia, SC

Leslie Fiore
Kentucky College of Business
Florence, KY

Diane Franks
National Career College
Tuscaloosa, AL

Tony Gabriel
Watterson College
Pasadena, CA

Karen Greer
Sawyer College
Merrillville, IN

Joyce Hill
Lansdale School of Business
North Wales, PA

Roxanne Hold
Excel College of Medical Arts
and Business
Madison, TN

Annette Jordan
Phillips Business College
Lynchburg, VA

Martha Juenke
American Medical Training
Institute
Miami, FL

Richard Krafcik
Sawyer College
Cleveland Heights, OH

Akeeboh Moore
CareerCom College of
Business
Oakland, CA

Basil Punsalan
Commonwealth College
Norfolk, VA

Alta Belle Roberts
Metro Business College
Rolla, MO

Sharon Adams
Sasser Sawyer College
Merrillville, IN

Joyce Shuey
Academy of Medical Arts and Business
Harrisburg, PA

Mary Ellen Stevenback
Lansdale School of Business
Harleysville, PA

Jinny Taylor
Academy of Medical Arts and Business
Harrisburg, PA

Edith Watts
Watterson College
Oxnard, CA

USING THE REVISED MEDICAL ASSISTANT KIT

The 10 anatomy and physiology books form the basis for a one-, two- or three-term introduction to body structure and function and human disease. Each book stands alone and may be used in the most appropriate sequence for your program.

Laboratory Processes for Medical Assisting and *Clinical Processes for Medical Assisting* can supplement the anatomy and physiology books as lab sections or they can be offered as separate courses.

We hope instructors and students alike will find a certain new clarity and precision in this new edition of the REGENTS/PRENTICE HALL MEDICAL ASSISTANT KIT. We look forward to your comments.

Mark Hartman
Editor, Health Professions

The Language of Medicine

Some of the words in this text will probably be new to you. They may seem very long and hard to remember. However, they will be easier to learn and understand if you know that they are made up of words or parts of words that come from Greek or Latin. As you begin to learn what these word parts mean, the names of muscles, bones, and diseases will begin to make sense to you.

First, there are words or parts of words that tell where a body part is in relation to other body parts. That is, they tell you about *location*. Here location. Here is a list of some location words:

Anterior	in front of
Distal	farthest from the center
Dorsal	at back
External	exterior, outside
Inferior	beneath or below
Internal	inside or inner part
Lateral	at side
Medial	at or near the midline of the body
Posterior	toward the back
Proximal	nearest to the center
Superior	over or above
Ventral	(in humans) front

Prefixes (part of words that come at the beginning of a word) that tell about location include:

ab-	away from
ad-	toward
endo-	inside, inner
epi-	upon
ex-	out of, away from
inter-	between

Next, there are parts of words that tell you how much or how big—about *quantity*. Here are some of them:

bi-	two
hemi-	half
mega-	great, large
mono-	one
multi-	many
poly-	many
quadri-	four
tetra-	four
tri-	three

There are also word parts that may come either at the end or the beginning of a word that can tell about the condition of a body part. Some of these are:

-algia	painful
dys-	improper, bad
-itis	inflammation
mal-	ill, bad
-sis	state or condition
ortho-	straight, normal, correct

Other parts of medical words may simply give the Greek or Latin name of a body part, or tell about its color or what it looks like. Some of the word parts that you will find in this book are listed here:

arthro	joint	*myo*	muscle
articulo	joint	*odont*	tooth
brachio	arm	*oid*	resembling
calc	(1) stone, (2) heel	*oma*	tumor
chondr	cartilage	*or*	mouth
cortic	outer layer	*orb*	circle
cune	wedge	*osteo*	bone
cyte	cell	*os*	bone
erythro	red	*poie*	make or produce
hemo	blood	*sarc*	flesh
form	shape	*sclero*	hard
lig	tie or bind	*spondylo*	spine

When these pieces are put together, they can describe body parts or conditions. (Sometimes vowels like *a*, *i*, or *o* may be added between the word parts, and sometimes a vowel may be dropped.) The words made of these pieces usually take the place of several nonmedical words. Here are some examples:

arthr + itis = joint inflammation
cune + i + form = wedge-shaped
erythro + cyte = red (blood) cell
hemo + poie + sis = condition of producing blood
odont + oid = shaped like a tooth
osteo + cyte = bone cell
oste + oma = bone tumor

You should be able to find and understand many others as you read this text. And checking a good medical dictionary will help you understand even more of the language of medicine.

CHAPTER 1

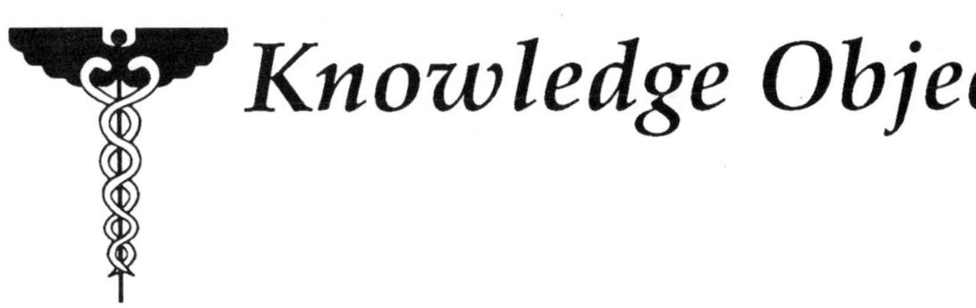

Knowledge Objectives

After completing this chapter, you should be able to:

Skeletal System Functions

- name five necessary functions of the musculoskeletal system
- describe the composition of bone tissue
- describe the haversian system and discuss its purpose and function
- list the parts and functions of bone marrow
- name three kinds of cartilage, list where they are found, and name a function of each

Bone Structure

- name four bone shapes and give an example of where each is found

Bone Formation and Maintenance

- describe how bone is formed

Specific Bones

- name and locate the bones of the skull
- name and locate the facial bones
- name the five regions of the vertebral column and list the number of bones found in each section
- define *kyphosis*, *lordosis*, and *scoliosis*
- give the number of true and false ribs
- locate the sternum and identify its three main parts
- list the differences between the axial and appendicular divisions of the skeleton
- locate and name the bones of the:
    - shoulder girdle
    - arm, wrist, and hand
    - pelvic girdle
    - leg, ankle, and foot

Articulations

- describe the two types of joints
- describe six types of movable joints

CHAPTER 1

The Skeletal System

INTRODUCTION

The musculoskeletal system has two parts: the bones that comprise the skeleton, and the muscles that are attached to them. The branch of medicine concerned with treating this system is called **orthopedics (OR thuh PEED icks)**. There are 206 named bones in the human body, and more than 600 skeletal muscles. These bones and muscles work together to perform five necessary functions.

1. **Movement** of the body and its parts, which is sometimes called *work*;
2. **Support and protection** of the organs and other systems of the body;
3. **Manufacture of blood** (or **hemopoiesis, HEE moh poy EE sis)**, which takes place in the red bone marrow;
4. **Storage of minerals,** such as calcium and phosphorus, in the bones, and of glycogen, a form of carbohydrate, in the muscles; and
5. **Generation of body heat,** a by-product of muscle contraction.

The voluntary muscles, those muscles that can be controlled by conscious effort, and the skeleton are usually considered a single system. This is because they interact closely. The simplest way for you to study this system is first to look at the two parts, both separately and as they work together, and then to learn about what kinds of diseases and other problems can occur in the system.

Functions of the Skeleton System

The skeleton is the part of the body that lasts the longest. Long after the soft tissues have disintegrated and disappeared, the skeleton remains—the structure of what was once a living creature. Scientists have learned a great deal about the human body through the study of the bones. When properly assembled, the skeleton is the supporting framework for the entire body. The skeleton also has several other less obvious functions.

The first of these is protection. The skull bones, the ribs, and the breastbone, for example example, shelter vital organs such as the brain, the lungs, and the heart from blows that might come from the outside. These bones are extremely strong, as anyone who has played contact sports can testify. But they are not completely invulnerable. Sometimes the skull is fractured, or a rib may be broken and may even puncture the lung it is designed to protect.

Another function of the skeleton is movement. Without a bony frame, the muscles would have difficulty causing an arm to swing, a fist to form, or a leg to take a forward step.

The other functions of the skeleton can-

- 206 NAMED BONES IN THE HUMAN BODY & MORE THAN 600 SKELETAL MUSCLES.
- FIVE NECESSARY FUNCTIONS: 1 MOVEMENT OF THE BODY AND ITS PARTS (WORK)

MUSCULOSKELETAL SYSTEM (PT 2)

BONES THAT COMPRISE THE SKELETON → MUSCLES ATTACHED TO THEM

ORTHOPEDICS -- THE BRANCH OF MEDICINE CONCERNED W/TREATING THIS SYSTEM

- SKELETON LASTS THE LONGEST OF ALL BODY PARTS.
  - SUPPORTED FRAMEWORK OF BODY.

2 SUPPORT & PROTECTION OF THE ORGANS AND OTHER SYSTEMS OF THE BODY

3. MANUFACTURE OF BLOOD (OR HEMOPOIESIS) WHICH TAKES PLACE IN THE RED BONE MARROW.

4 STORAGE OF MINERALS, SUCH AS CALCIUM AND PHOSPHORUS, IN THE BONES, AND OF GLYCOGEN, A FORM OF CARBOHYDRATE IN THE MUSCLES.

5 GENERATION OF BODY HEAT, A BY PRODUCT OF MUSCLE CONTRACTION.

not be seen or even felt. They take place inside the bones, as part of the interlocking systems that keep the body alive. One of these functions of the skeleton is producing, maintaining, and repairing itself. The cells and tissues that make up the skeleton continually create new cells and new bone as the old ones wear out, become injured, or break down. The same process also affects the level of calcium in the blood, which in turn affects other functions of the muscles, the nerves, and the digestive system. Finally, the bones encase the marrow, where most of the blood cells (the red cells that carry oxygen, the white cells that protect against infection, and the platelets) are manufactured through a process known as **hemopoiesis**.

Before studying the names of the bones, it is important for you to understand what the bones are made of, how they are made, and how they function. This will help you in understanding diseases and injuries of the bones, and in assisting in their treatment.

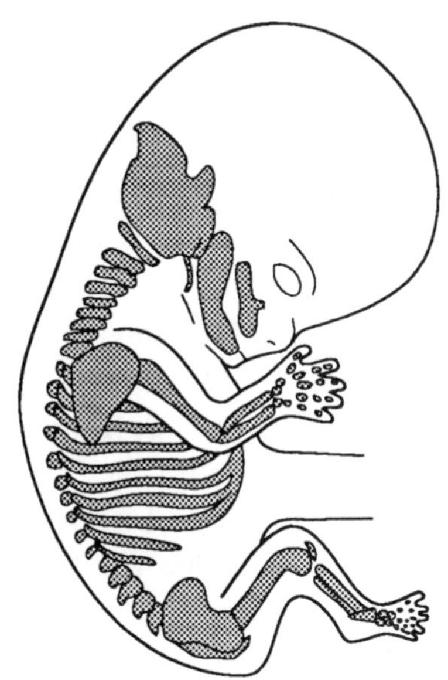

Figure 1: The cartilagenous fetal skeleton at age 7 weeks.

Bone Tissue

Skeletal formation begins early in fetal life. By age 7 weeks, most of the skeletal system has been formed, although at this point it consists entirely of flexible cartilage (see Figure 1). This flexibility is vital during childbirth, and later it protects the child from injury from the many falls and spills that occur during infancy and toddlerhood.

The bones of an adult seem to be solid and passive, but in fact blood vessels carry blood through them, blood cells are manufactured in them, and they have a complex structure. Human bones are of different shapes, sizes, and weights, depending on where they are in the body and how they are used. For example, a long bone (see Figure 2) in an arm or leg has **compact,** or dense, **bone** (also called **cortex (KOR tecks)**) along its length for extra strength and rigidity, and **cancellous (KAN se lus)**, or spongy, **bone** at the ends for growth and flexibility. Under a microscope, compact bone has few apparent pores, while cancellous bone looks like latticework.

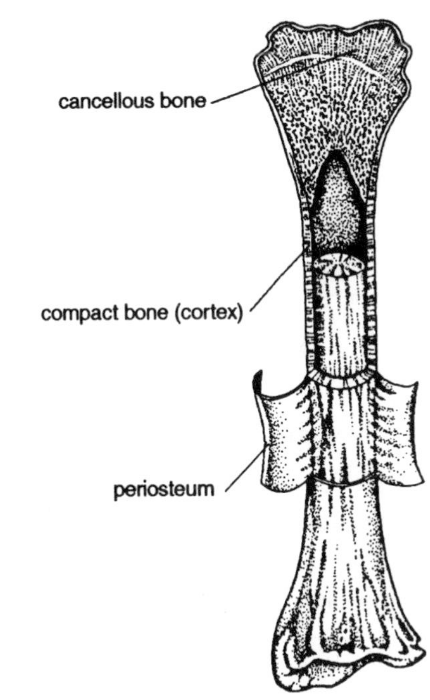

Figure 2: Typical long bone.

Bone Matrix. Nonliving material known as **bone matrix** (MAY tricks) is the basic tissue of bone. It is made up mainly of fluids and collagen, a protein. Collagen becomes a kind of gelatin when it is boiled, which is why chicken broth made from boiled chicken bones will jell in the refrigerator. Collagen is also a major ingredient in connective tissues, such as ligaments, tendons, and cartilage. It is the most common protein in the human body.

The bone matrix is hard because it is saturated with mineral salts. Calcium phosphate is the most important of these mineral salts. These minerals provide about two-thirds of the weight of bone. The process of hardening that occurs when calcium and other minerals are deposited in bone matrix is called calcification or ossification. Without the hardening mineral salts, bone is so flexible and elastic that it can be tied in a knot. The minerals that make bone hard or rigid are deposited into the bone matrix in thin, hard layers. These layers, called **lamellae** (lah MEL ee), are arranged in different patterns, depending on what type of bone they form.

Living bone cells called **osteocytes (OS tee oh SYTE)** are interspersed within this structure (see Figure 3). They are protected by the hard layers of lamellae. The microscopic openings where the osteocytes are found are called **lacunae (lah KEW nee).** The lacunae are filled with bone matrix fluid. Osteocytes help develop and maintain bone tissue. If these living elements of bone are killed or removed, the bone becomes brittle and is crushed easily. The osteocytes are themselves maintained in one of two ways. In cancellous bone, blood vessels pass through the lattice-like columns of the bone matrix. In compact bone, the cells are nourished through a more complex arrangement called the **haversian (huh VUR zhun) systems**. These haversian systems can be seen with the help of a powerful microscope.

Haversian Systems. A **haversian system** (see Figure 3) is the structural unit of compact bone tissue. It is named after an English physician, Clopton Havers, who studied and described the structure of bone in the late 1600s. The function of the haversian system is to supply nutrients to and remove wastes from the osteocytes through a system of canals. These canals allow veins, arteries, and lymph vessels to penetrate the bone matrix. There are four kinds of canals and passageways in the system.

The first ones are **Volkmann's canals,** which enter the bone matrix from the outside. If the **periosteum (PERR ee OS tee um)** or outer membrane, were stripped off a living bone, tiny bleeding points would appear. These are Volkmann's canals, and through them microscopic veins and arteries penetrate the bone. The second ones are the haversian canals, which extend throughout compact bone and make passageways for the blood vessels to reach the individual bone cells. Each of the haversian canals is surrounded by circular layers of thin, flat sheets of bone matrix called lamellae. Between them run even smaller passageways called **canaliculi (KAN uh LICK yoo lye),** the third kind of canal in the system. Canaliculi carry nutrients and wastes between the vessels in the haversian canals and the cells themselves. The cells are surrounded by fluid-filled spaces called lacunae which literally means cavities. These are the fourth type of passageway in the system. In the lacunae, the actual transfer of nutrients and wastes finally occurs. The wastes are carried away from the cells through the veins in the system, and the arteries carry nutrients into the bone.

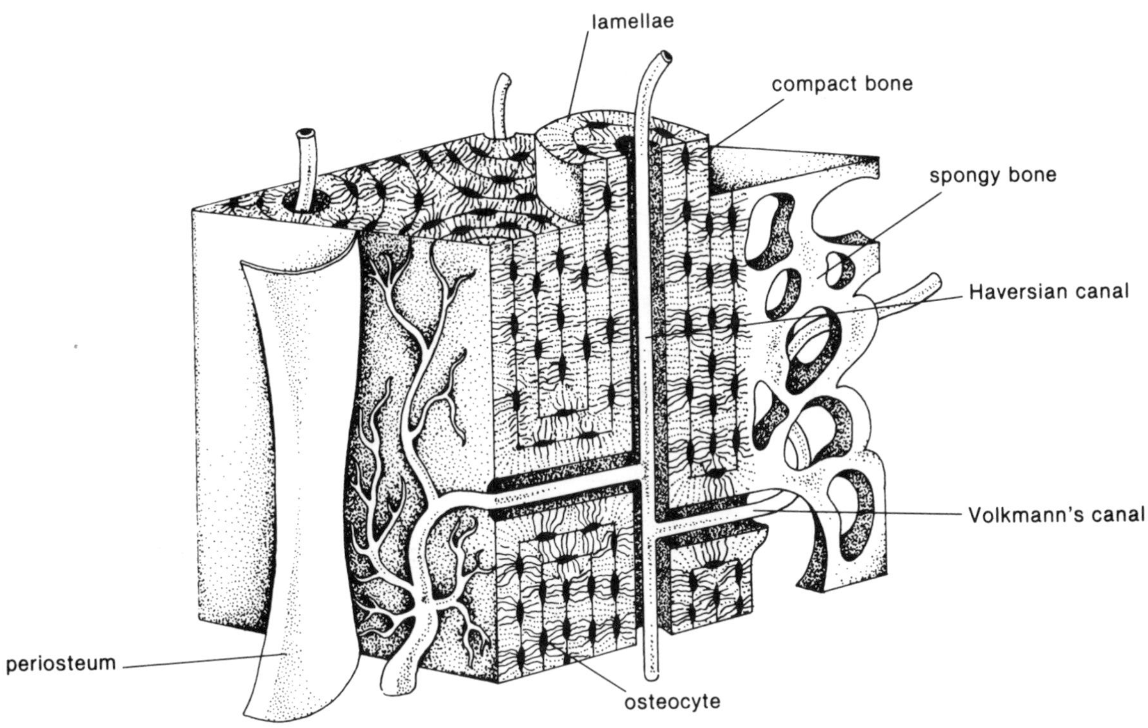

Figure 3: Haversian canal systems.

Bone Marrow. **Bone marrow** is another structural component of bone. There are two kinds of marrow, red and yellow. **Red marrow** is made up of connective tissue, blood vessels, and several kinds of cells that manufacture red and white blood cells. (The process of making these cells is called hemopoiesis. From birth through early childhood, all bone marrow is red. As a person becomes older, the need for blood cell production decreases and some red marrow is converted into yellow marrow. In adults, red marrow is found in the cancellous bone in the long bones of the arms and legs, and in other bones such as the ribs, breastbone, and vertebrae. In newborn babies and children, who are growing and need increasing amounts of blood cells, red marrow occurs in many more bones. It becomes yellow marrow as the demand for blood cells decreases.

Yellow marrow is also made up of connective tissue, blood vessels, and cells. Some of the cells make white blood cells, but most of them are fat cells. Yellow marrow occurs mostly in the central core of the long bones, but small amounts of it also are found in the haversian canals.

Cartilage

Cartilage (KAHR ti lij) tissue is considered part of the skeleton because most of it is attached directly to the bones. The main difference between cartilage and bone is that cartilage contains no calcium phosphate and therefore it is not hard or rigid. Cartilage serves as connective tissue between bones. It is tough and strong, but also flexible enough to allow movement. Another difference between bone and cartilage is that cartilage has no blood vessels or canals, because it is not nourished in the same way as bone.

There are three kinds of cartilage: **hyaline (HYE uh lin), elastic,** and **fibrous.** Most of the cartilage in the human body is the type called hyaline. It looks shiny, and is made up of a few cells in a network of col-

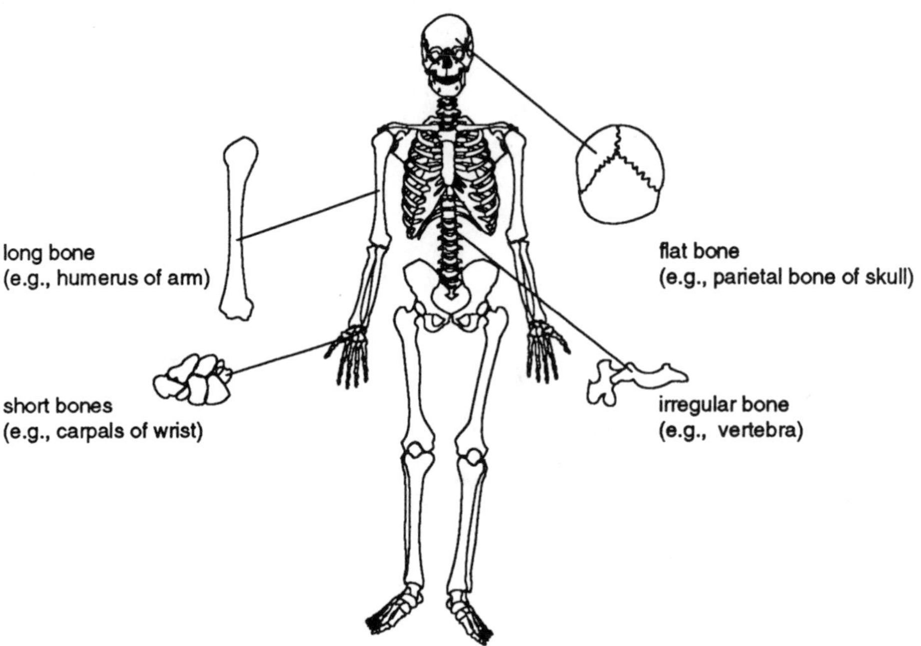

Figure 4: Types of bone are classified by shape.

lagenous fibers; that is, fibers made of collagen. Hyaline cartilage covers the ends of bones at the joints, where it is called **articular cartilage,** and the ends of the ribs where they attach to the sternum, or breastbone. These rib cartilages are called **costal cartilages,** after the Latin name for rib, which is *costa.* Since they are an essential part of the skeleton, articular and costal cartilages together are sometimes called skeletal cartilage.

Hyaline cartilage also occurs in other body structures, such as the nose, larynx (voice box), trachea (windpipe), and bronchial tubes. Hyaline cartilage, in an embryo or fetus, later develops into bone.

Elastic cartilage, as its name implies, is more flexible than the other two types. Instead of collagenous fibers, it is made up mostly of elastic fibers. In the human body the outer ear, the eustachian tube, and some parts of the larynx are made of elastic cartilage.

The third type of cartilage is known as fibrous or **fibrocartilage.** Its main function is to connect the skeletal bones. The vertebral discs in the spine are made of this kind of cartilage. Fibrocartilage usually attaches to hyaline cartilage at the point where the bones join. It provides a strong link because it is somewhat rigid, and it meshes with the skeletal cartilage tightly so that the two substances are essentially continuous.

Two other parts of the musculoskeletal system, tendons and ligaments, are described in the section on the joints. (STOP AND REVIEW, page 9.)

Bone Structure

Once you understand the microscopic view of the skeletal system, you can begin to look at individual bones. They come in four shapes: long, short, flat and irregular (see Figure 4). Short, flat, and irregular bones have the same basic structure—spongy or cancellous bone in the center, and compact bone on the outside. The lacunae in the center portion usually are filled with red marrow. For an idea of which bones are classified under which shape, see Table 1.

Long bones have a more complex and also a more predictable structure than the

STOP AND REVIEW

1. Approximately how many bones are found in the mature adult body?
2. Approximately how many muscles are found in the body?
3. What is the branch of medicine concerned with treating the musculoskeletal system?
4. Name five functions of the musculoskeletal system.
   a. ______________________
   b. ______________________
   c. ______________________
   d. ______________________
   e. ______________________
5. Name two kinds of bone tissue.
   a. ______________________
   b. ______________________
6. Name the two major components of bone matrix.
   a. ______________________
   b. ______________________
7. The substance that makes bone hard is ______________________ .
8. Another name for the process of bone hardening is ______________________ .
9. Osteocytes in compact bone receive blood and nourishment through what system?
10. Describe the structure, location, and function of:
    a. red marrow ______________________
    b. yellow marrow ______________________
11. Name two differences between the structures of bone and cartilage.
    a. ______________________
    b. ______________________
12. Match the type of cartilage with its characteristic, the body part in which it is found, or the function it performs.

a. hyaline	____ 1. covers ends of bones at joints
b. elastic	____ 2. found in the larynx
c. fibrous	____ 3. found in the embryo
	____ 4. made up of collagenous fibers
	____ 5. found in vertebral discs
	____ 6. attaches to hyaline cartilage where bones join
	____ 7. found in outer ear
	____ 8. made up of elastic fibers
	____ 9. somewhat rigid

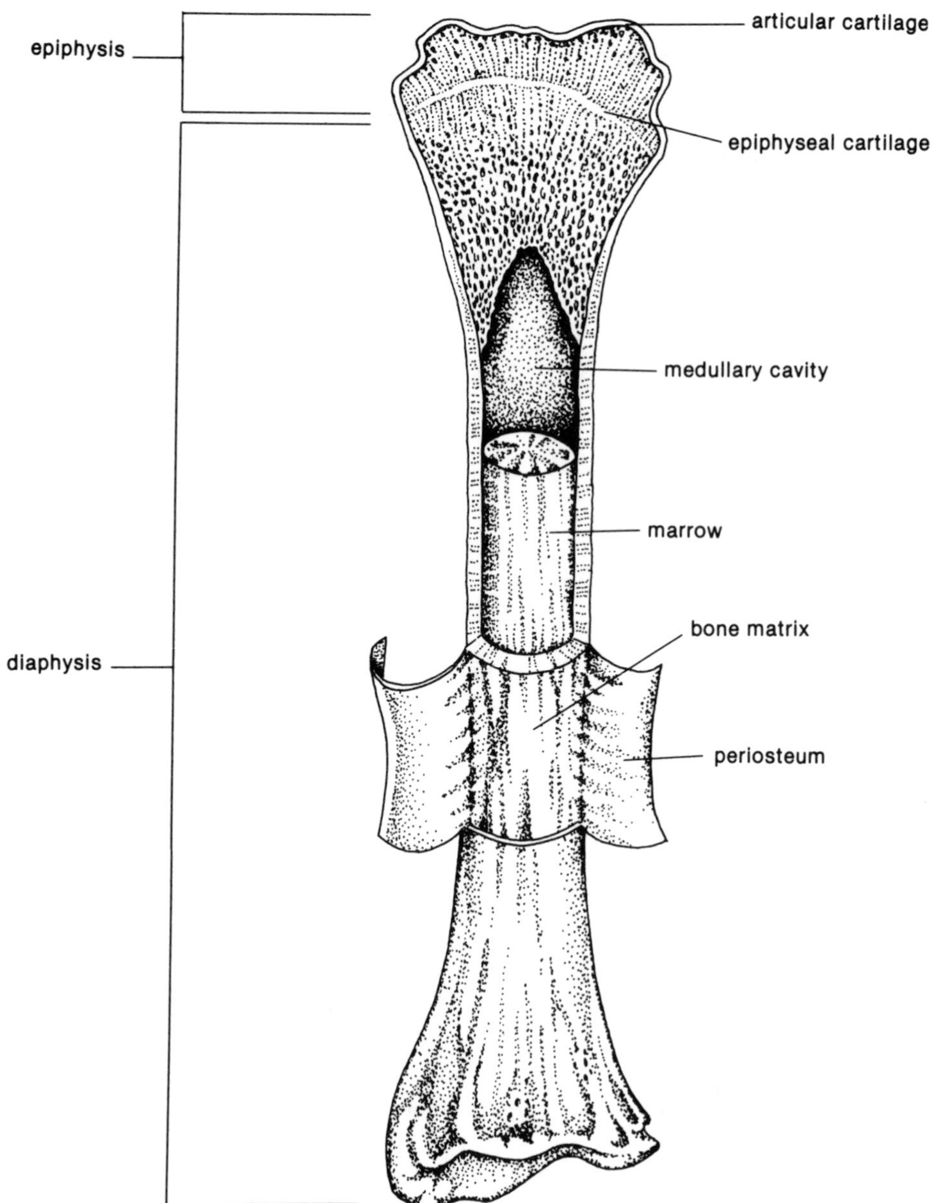

Figure 5: Components of long bone.

other three shapes. By looking at the parts of a long bone, as they are shown in Figure 5, you can better understand how all the tissues and structures function in a living bone.

Each long bone, regardless of its size, has the following components:

- Articular cartilage (hyaline) at one or both ends;
- Cancellous (spongy) bone tissue, also at each end, attached to the cartilage;
- Compact bone tissue in the form of a tube along the shaft (bone matrix);
- A space inside the tube that is filled with yellow marrow and lined with cancellous bone and red marrow;
- An outside covering that extends to the cartilage at each end.

Each of these elements of long bone has a purpose. The cartilage at the ends is a tough but flexible cushion for the joint, so that the bone can be moved with a minimum of wear. The cancellous, or spongy, bone is the site for bone growth. It also gives structural strength near the joint, where the bone is

Table 1: Examples of Bone Types

Long Bones	Short Bones	Flat Bones	Irregular Bones
humerus, ulna (arms), femur, tibia, fibula (leg), phalanges (fingers and toes)	carpals (wrists), tarsals (ankles)	frontal, parietal (top of head), ribs, scapulae (shoulders)	vertebrae, sacrum, coccyx (neck, back), sphenoid, ethmoid, mandible (face)

often under strain. The cancellous bone also contains red marrow, which makes blood cells. Compact tissue strengthens the shaft because of its density, and provides a network for blood vessels through the haversian canals. In the core, the yellow marrow makes white blood cells and stores fat.

The shaft of the long bone is technically known as the **diaphysis (dye AF ih sis)**. The areas of cancellous bone where growth occurs are called **epiphyses (eh PIF ih sis)**. The core is called the **medullary (MED yoo LERR ee) cavity.** The outer covering is the periosteum (see Figure 5). (STOP AND REVIEW, page 12.)

How Bone is Made and Maintained

Before a child is born, the process of **ossification (OS ih fih KAY shun)** or bone formation, begins. In the early stages of development, either membrane or cartilage forms where the bones will be. Then these tissues gradually change into bone. The process is different depending on whether the original material is membrane or cartilage.

The cranium, or skull, is an example of bone formed from membrane. In this process, the membrane becomes the periosteum, or outer covering of the bone. The membrane is made of fibrous tissue with **osteoblasts (OS tee oh BLASTS),** or bone-forming cells, in the center. It is full of a network of blood vessels. As bone begins to form, tiny, needle-like objects called *spicules* appear in the center of the potential bone. Then collagenous fibers appear, and granules of calcium and other minerals begin to be deposited in those fibers. The fibers begin to form into columns of calcified tissue, and the osteoblasts become osteocytes (living bone cells) in the spaces between the columns. Spicules continue to form along the outside of the bony tissue, and layer after layer of calcified fiber is added to the structure until the bone is formed.

The formation of long bones begins instead with rods of cartilage in roughly the shape and position of the future bone. These rods are covered with membrane. Ossification begins in the center and ends of the shaft, at ossification centers. The extreme ends of the bones remain as cartilage, in some cases until adulthood. This cartilage is called **epiphyseal (EP ih FIZ ee ul) cartilage.**

Cartilage ossification involves two processes that occur simultaneously. On the outside of the bone, the membrane goes through the process described above and forms the periosteum and a hard outer layer for the bone. At the same time, the cartilage cells at the ossification centers begin to arrange themselves in rows. These cells gradually become separated from each other and from any sources of nourishment by deposits of calcium made in the surrounding tissues. The cartilage cells die, leaving empty spaces between the calcium layer.

As these spaces appear, blood vessels and osteoblasts move to the ossification centers from the outside layer of bone at the periosteum. The osteoblasts begin to add layers of calcified tissue around the ossifica-

STOP AND REVIEW

1. Name the four types of bone based on shape.

   a. ____________________

   b. ____________________

   c. ____________________

   d. ____________________

2. Cancellous bone in the center and compact bone on the outside describes what bone type(s)? ____________________

3. Match the shapes of bones with the parts of the body in which they are found. (Each answer may be used more than once.)

a. long	____ 1. top of head
b. short	____ 2. arm
c. flat	____ 3. face
d. irregular	____ 4. ankle
	____ 5. chest
	____ 6. neck
	____ 7. foot
	____ 8. ear

4. Match the parts of a long bone with their function. (Each may be used more than once.)

a. cartilage	____ 1. cushions joints
b. cancellous bone	____ 2. site of bone growth
c. compact bone	____ 3. gives extra strength
d. red marrow	____ 4. contains red marrow
e. yellow marrow	____ 5. adds density
f. medullary cavity	____ 6. contains haversian canals
	____ 7. stores fat
	____ 8. makes white blood cells
	____ 9. makes red blood cells
	____ 10. adds flexibility

tion centers to strengthen the walls of the bone. They eventually become osteocytes. At the same time, **osteoclasts (OS tee oh KLASTS)**, or bone-destroying cells, appear in the middle of the bone structure. These cells create a central cavity in the bone called the **medullary (MED eh LER ee) cavity.** This is where the central core of bone marrow is deposited in the long bones.

The osteoblasts continue to create bone tissue and the osteoclasts continue to destroy it until the medullary cavity is formed and the layers of cancellous bone, compact bone, and periosteum are established. The process still continues, but at a slower rate as the bones grow. The osteoclasts destroy the bone cells around the core of the bone. This enlarges the space for the marrow. At the same time, the osteoblasts continue to create bony tissue and osteocytes at the outside of the bone beneath the periosteum, and at each end in the epiphyseal cartilages.

For ossification to proceed normally, the body must have an adequate intake of dietary calcium. This mineral is found in dairy foods, canned salmon, and green vegetables such as broccoli.

In short, when a person is growing, the bone-forming cells called osteoblasts continually lay down layers of calcium on the outside of the bone at the same time as bone-destroying cells called osteoclasts are eating away at the center of the bone. This continual eating away on the inside and building up on the outside of the bone causes the medullary central cavity to enlarge.

In adulthood the process almost stops, and the bones stay about the same size and shape. However, inactive osteoblasts remain in the bone under the periosteum. They are activated to repair the bone when an injury such as a fracture occurs. In old age, the osteoclasts may become more active than the osteoblasts. If this happens, the bones will become increasingly light and brittle as the central core enlarges and the outer structure is not replenished.

This process of ossification cannot take place without the proper level of calcium in the blood stream. The balance is maintained through the action of a hormone called **parathormone (PAR uh THOR mone).**

Bone and Calcium Balance. Parathormone, or parathyroid hormone, is made by the parathyroid glands. There are four of these glands, and they are located on the back surface of the thyroid gland in the neck. When parathormone is released, it stimulates the osteoclasts to increase the breaking down, or resorption, of bone tissue.

As the bone tissue is broken down, calcium and phosphates enter the blood stream. Parathormone causes the kidneys to selectively filter out the phosphates but not the calcium. This leads to an increase in calcium in the blood. The phosphates that are filtered out are excreted with the urine. If the hormone is not released, or if there is not enough calcium in the body, the level of calcium in the blood will drop below normal. The abnormally low calcium level in the blood can cause such things as muscle spasms and irregular blood clotting. It can also affect the process of digestion, the absorption of nutrients, and the disposal of wastes by the cells.

Vitamin D has the opposite effect to parathormone. This vitamin encourages the absorption of calcium from the blood stream into the bones, and stimulates the osteoblasts to form new bone. Vitamin D is found in fish oil, egg yolks, and fresh vegetables. It is also made by the body when sun rays come in contact with the skin.

This continuous cycle of breaking down old cells and replacing them with new ones maintains the right amount of calcium in the

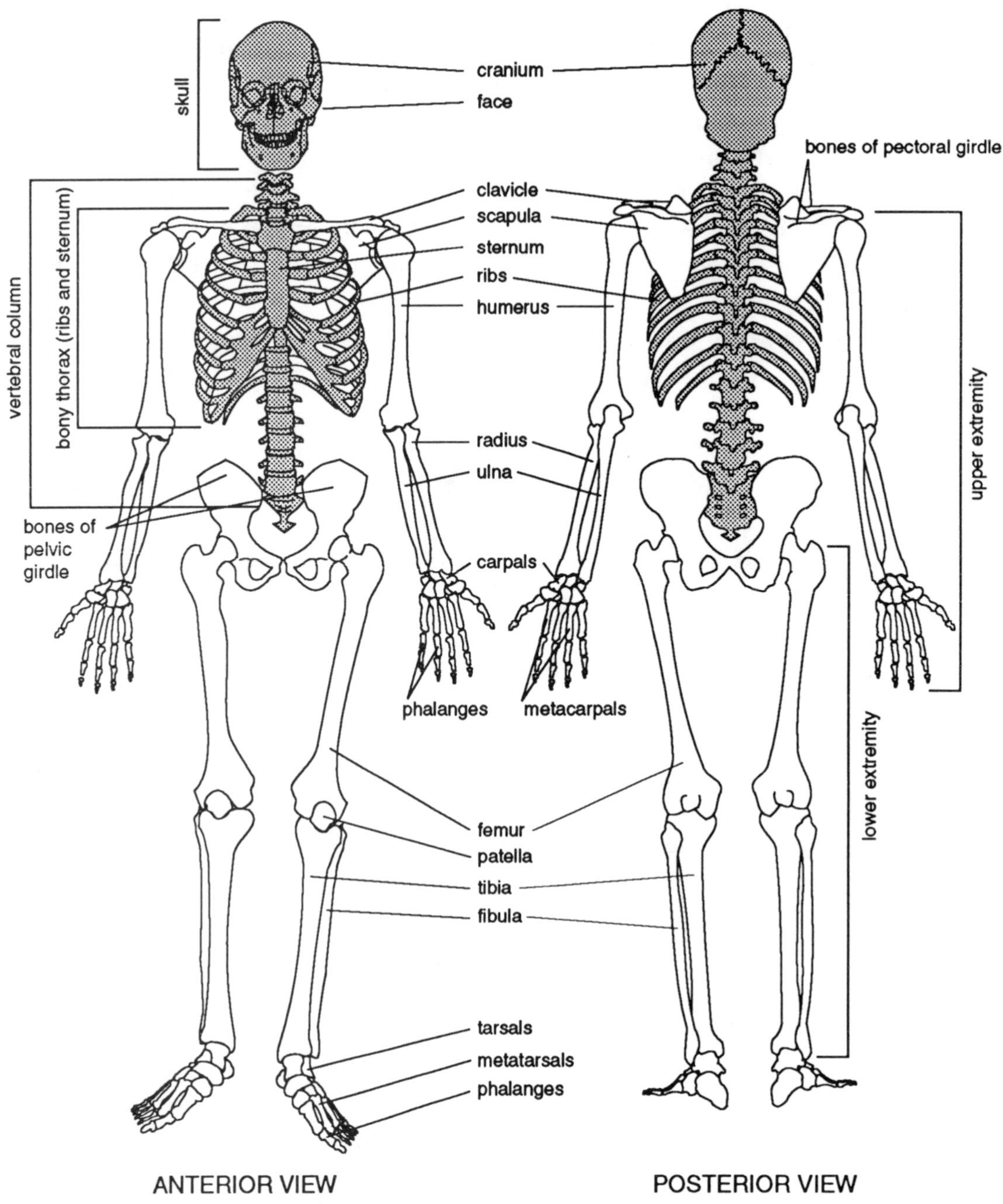

Figure 6: The human skeleton. The bones of the axial skeleton are shaded. The bones of the appendicular skeleton are not shaded.

blood, so that the whole body can function properly. If the balance of calcium and vitamin D is not maintained, the bones may become soft and bend too easily. The result may be bowleg and abnormally large joints. (See Osteomalacia in Chapter 3.) (STOP AND REVIEW, page 15.)

Specific Bones

There are 206 named bones in the normal adult human body. There are also some tiny bones (called sesamoid bones) that are imbedded in tendons and in the joints of the skull. Most of these are not named. The 206 major bones are divided into two groups

STOP AND REVIEW

1. Name two kinds of tissue in the fetus which eventually change into bone.

   a. ______________________________

   b. ______________________________

2. An example of a bone formed from membrane is the ______________________________

3. An example of a bone formed from cartilage is the ______________________________

4. Circle one: In old age, osteoclasts may be (more/less) active than osteoblasts.

5. Circle one: If (osteoclasts/osteoblasts) are more active, bone becomes brittle.

6. The proper level of calcium circulating in the blood is necessary for what bone process to take place?

7. Which types of bone are formed from the inside out?

   a. ______________________________

   b. ______________________________

   c. ______________________________

8. Match the definition with the word.

   a. osteoblast

   b. osteoclast

   c. osteocyte

   ____1. bone cell

   ____2. bone former

   ____3. bone destroyer

9. True/False: Parathormone stimulates the osteoblasts to form new bone.

10. Label the parts of the long bone shown in the diagram at right with the names listed below.

    marrow, bone matrix, articular cartilage, epiphyseal cartilage, periosteum, diaphysis, epiphysis, medullary cavity

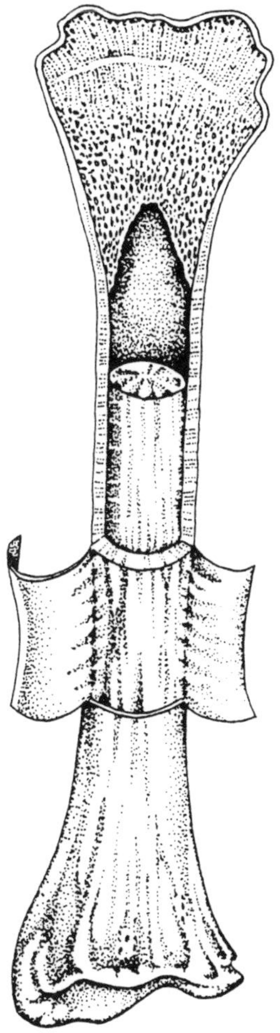

Table 2: Bone Groups

Axial Skeleton	*Number of Bones*
Skull	8
Face	14
Ear	6
Hyoid	1
Spine	26
Sternum and ribs (rib cage)	25
	80
Appendicular Skeleton	
Shoulders, arms, and hands	64
Hips, legs, and feet	62
	Total Bones 126

(see Figure 6): the **axial (ACK see ul)** skeleton, which includes the bones along the axis or center of the body; and the **appendicular (AP en DICK yoo lur)** skeleton, which consists of the limbs or appendages (see Table 2).

Cranium or Skull. The cranium, or skull (see Table 3), appears to be solid in an adult, but it is actually several flat bones joined together with immovable, rigid **articulations (ahr TICK yoo LAY schunz)** or joints called

Table 3: Bones of the Cranium or Skull

Frontal	forehead	1
Parietal	top and top of sides	2
Temporal	lower part of sides	2
Occipital	back	1
Ethoid	behind nose in eye sockets	1
Sphenoid	side and behind nose	2

sutures (SOO churz). They encase the brain in a hard shell that is very difficult to penetrate. In infants, however, the cranial bones are not completely formed and the sutures are not complete (see Figures 7 and 8). This allows the skull to compress somewhat during the birth process.

The "soft spots" between the cranial bones are called **fontanels (FON tuh nelz).** They gradually ossify and close up. The largest one is called the *frontal* or *anterior* (at the front) fontanel. It is located between the frontal bone and the parietal bone, and it is the last one to harden. It usually is closed up by the time a child is 18 months old. The others are called the posterior (rear), anterolateral (side front), and posterolateral (side rear) fontanels. The posterior fontanel is the

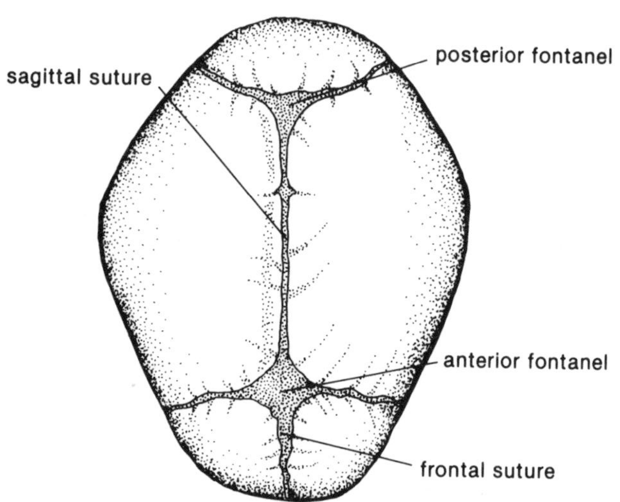

Figure 7: Superior view of fetal skull.

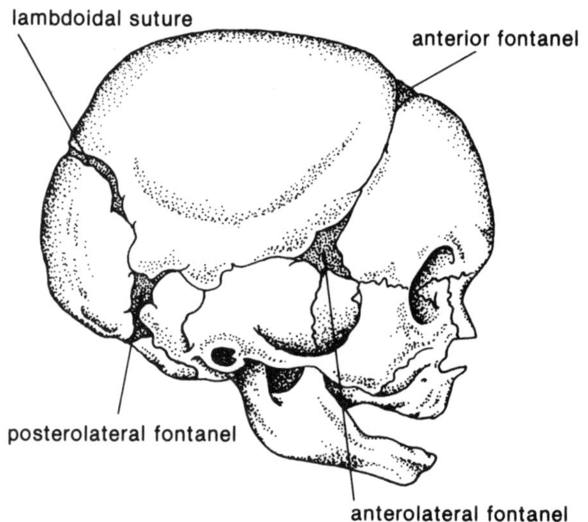

Figure 8: Lateral view of fetal skull.

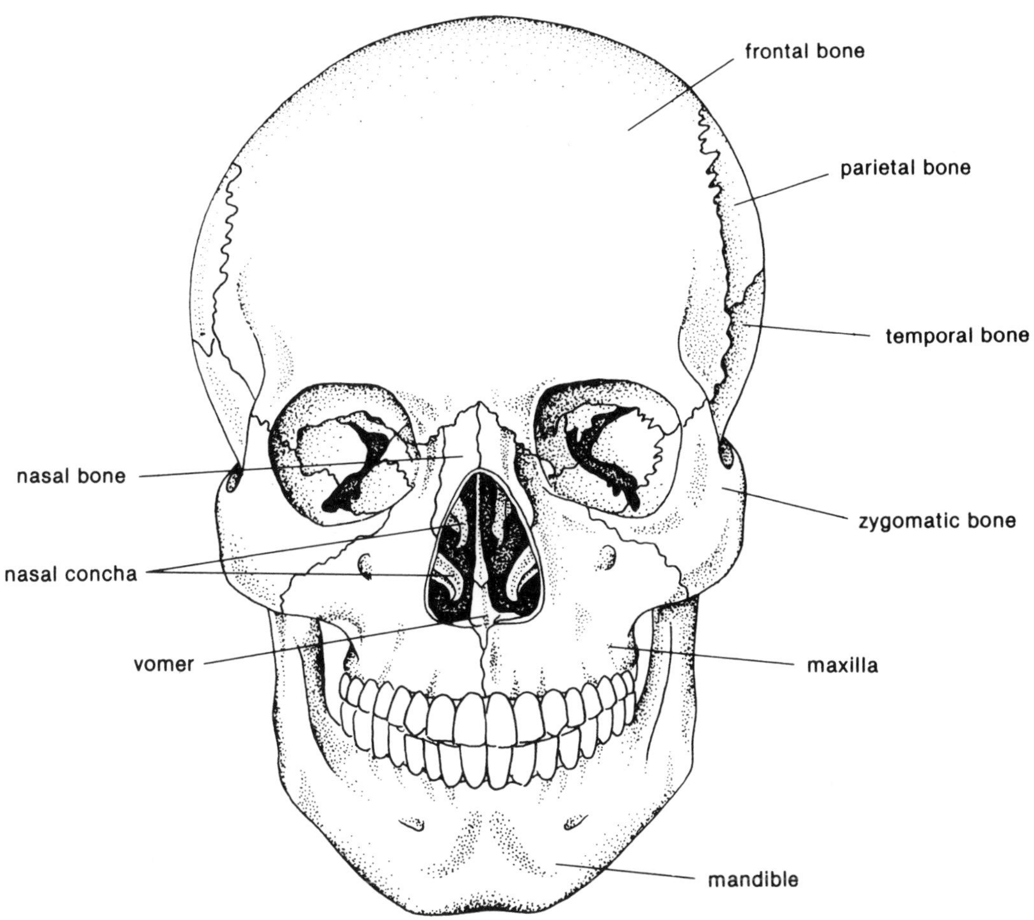

Figure 9: Anterior view of skull.

first to harden, becoming closed up by the second month.

The frontal bone forms the forehead. It extends from the top of the eye sockets to the top of the head. There it articulates with, or joins, the **parietal (pah RYE eh tul) bones,** which cover the back of the top of the head and extend to the sides. These bones form most of the roof and sides of the cranium (see Figures 9 and 10).

The two temporal bones join the parietal bones on each side of the head and extend to the base of the ear. The opening for the ear is in the temporal bone. It is called the **auditory meatus (AW di TOR ee me AY tus).** The **occipital (ock SIP ih tul) bone** covers the bottom of the head in the rear (see Figure 11). There is a large opening, or **foramen,** in the bottom of this bone, where the spinal column attaches to the skull. It is called the **foramen magnum (foh RAY mun MAG num),** which in Latin means *large opening.* There are 14 similar but smaller openings in the cranial bones, through which nerves and blood vessels pass.

Both the **ethmoid (ETH moyd) bone** and the **sphenoid (SFEE noyd) bone** are behind the eye sockets and the nose. The sphenoid has two wing-like projections, which hold all the other cranial bones except the temporal bones in place. On the upper surface of the sphenoid there is a depression called the **sella turcica (SEL uh TUR sih kuh)** which holds the pituitary gland. The ethmoid bone is located behind the nasal bones and in front of the sphenoid (see Figure 12).

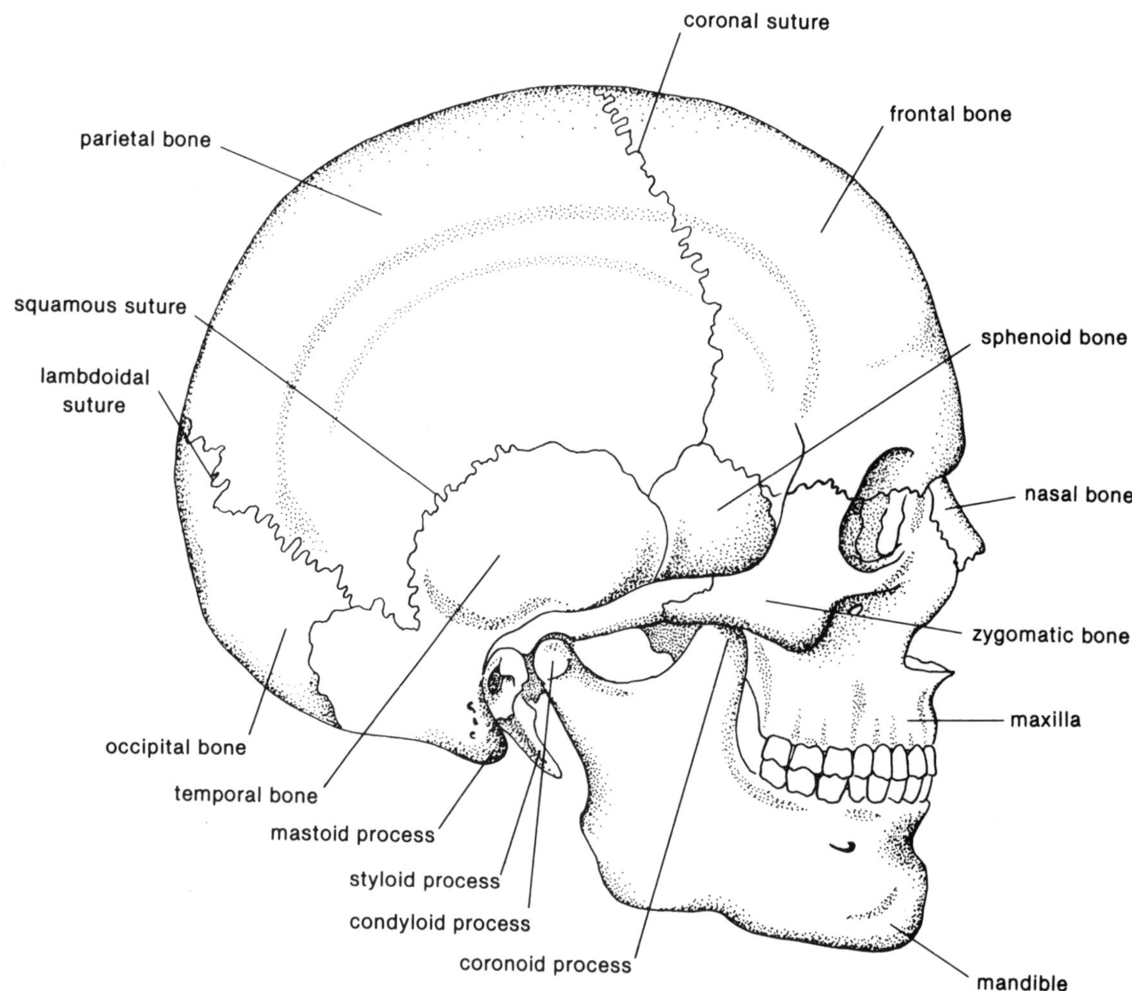

Figure 10: Lateral view of skull.

Facial Bones. The facial bones (see Table 4) are located in the anterior, or front, of the cranium. They are irregular bones that protect the sense organs, such as the eyes and nose, and form the shape of the face (see Figure 10).

Table 4: Facial Bones

Maxilla	upper jaw	2
Zygomatic	cheek bone	2
Nasal	bridge of nose	2
Mandible	lower jaw	1
Lacrimal	in eye sockets	2
Palatine	roof of mouth	2
Concha	in nasal passage	3
Vomer	base and rear of nasal passage	1

The two **maxillae (mack SIL ee)** and the **mandible (MAN dih bul)** together form the mouth. The maxillae articulate in the center of the face and are the same shape, while the mandible is a single bone that forms the jaw line and chin. The **nasal bones** are also two symmetrical bones, which join in the center to form the bridge of the nose, and attach to the top of the maxillae. The two **zygomatic (ZYE go MAT ick) bones** attach to the sides of each maxilla and form the lower edge of the edge of the eye sockets (see Figure 11). Each zygomatic bone curves outward in the zygomatic arch, which shapes the line of the cheek.

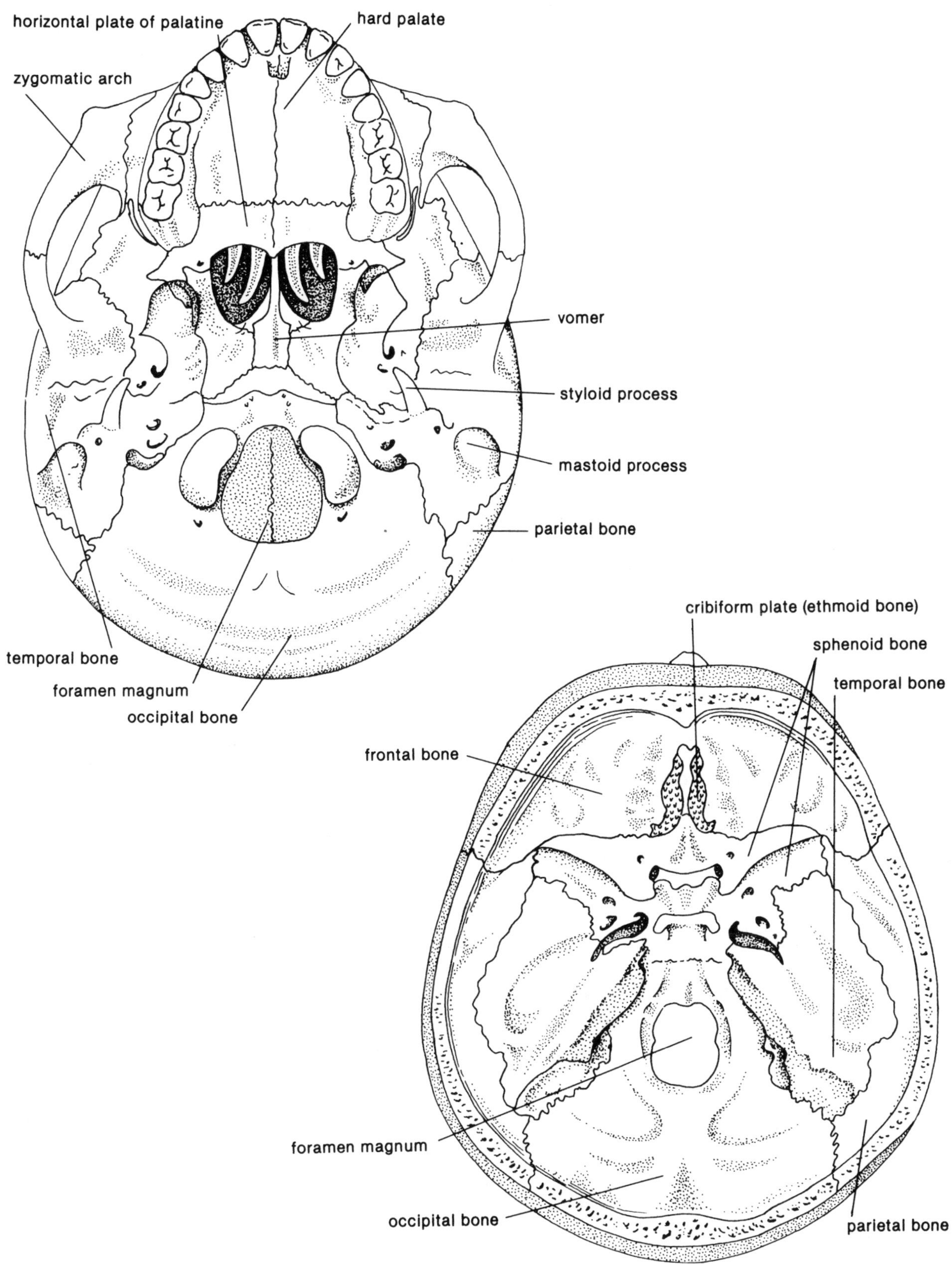

Figure 11: Basal view of skull.

Figure 12: Superior view of skull.

STOP AND REVIEW

1. Approximately how many bones are found in the mature adult body? ________________
2. True/False: An infant's skull is completely ossified at birth.
3. List the bones that are found in the axial skeleton. ________________________________

   ____
4. Articulation is another word for ____ .
5. Name the two major fontanels found in the infant skull.
   a. ____
   b. ____
6. Two other fontanels which may be present in the infant skull are the:
   a. ____
   b. ____
7. Rigid joints found in the skull are called ________________________________ .
8. The large opening in the skull through which the spinal column attaches is called the

   ____
9. The auditory meatus in the temporal bone is the opening for the ____________________

   ____ .
10. Circle the correct answer.

    The sphenoid bone:
    a. joins the parietal bones on each side of the head
    b. contains the opening for the ear
    c. holds almost all the other cranial bones in place
    d. is located behind the nasal bones

The two **lacrimal (LACK rih mul) bones** are inside the eye sockets along the side of the nose. They are named after the lacrimal ducts, or tear ducts, which are located at the inside corners of the eyes. The two **palatine (PAL uh tine) bones** are behind the part of the mouth called the hard palate, or roof. The superior, inferior, and middle **conchae (KONG kee)** are in the sides of the nasal passage. The **vomer (VOH mer)** forms the base of the nasal passage and the nasal septum, the wall between the nostrils.

The **sinuses,** which are part of the respiratory system, are cavities in the facial and cranial bones (see Figure 13). They are named the frontal, maxillary, ethmoidal, and sphenoidal sinuses after the bones in which they are found.

Hyoid Bone. The **hyoid (HYE oyd) bone** is located at the top of the neck between the mandible and the larynx, or voice box. It is

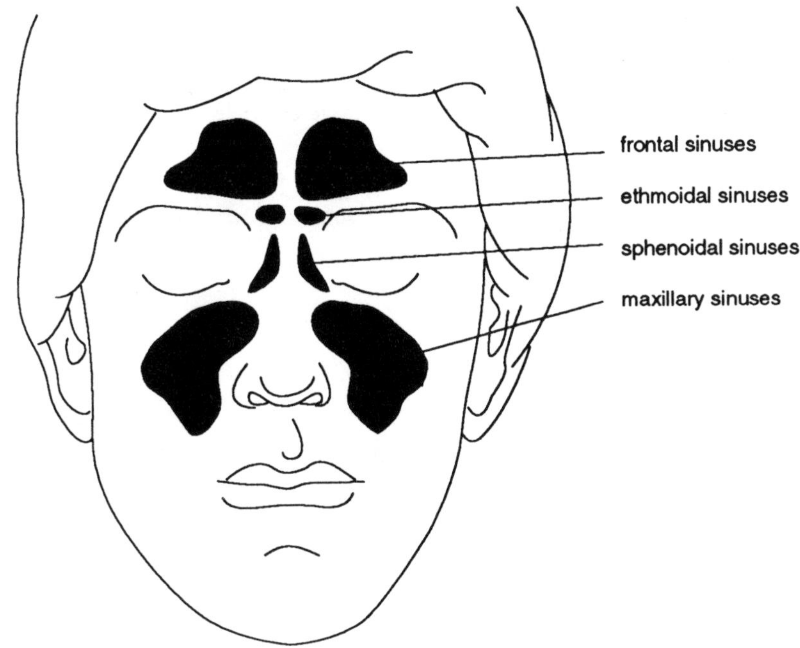

Figure 13: Frontal view of sinuses.

shaped like a "u." The hyoid bone is not connected by a joint to any other bone. Instead, it is suspended from the mandible and the temporal bones by ligaments. (STOP AND REVIEW, page 20.)

Vertebral Column. The **vertebrae (VUR teh bree)** (see Table 5) are stacked on each other to form a strong but flexible column with an opening through the center. The spinal cord, which is part of the nervous system and is linked directly to the base of the brain, is encased in and protected by this bony structure. Adults have a total of 26 bones in the spinal column. In children, however, the **sacrum (SAY krum)** has five bones and the **coccyx (KOCK sicks)** has four. These small bones gradually fuse together to form single bones. Before these small bones fuse, children have 33 spinal bones.

Each vertebra is separated and cushioned from the ones above and below it by disks of cartilage called intervertebral discs. The condition called hernaited or slipped disc or ruptured disk occurs when one of these pieces of cartilage moves sideways from its position between two bony vertebrae. The disk may then press on a nerve and cause pain or even paralysis.

The vertebrae (see Figure 14) are irregular bones that are the same general shape with variations depending on their locations. Each one has a central opening for the spinal cord to pass through, and several **processes,** or projections (see Figure 15). The process at the top of each vertebra (along the

Table 5: Vertebral Column

Vertebrae	Number of vertebrae in a child	Number of vertebrae in an adult
Cervical (in neck)	7	7
Thoracic (in chest area)	12	12
Lumbar (in lower back)	5	5
Sacrum (base of spine)	5	1
Coccyx (tail bone)	4	1

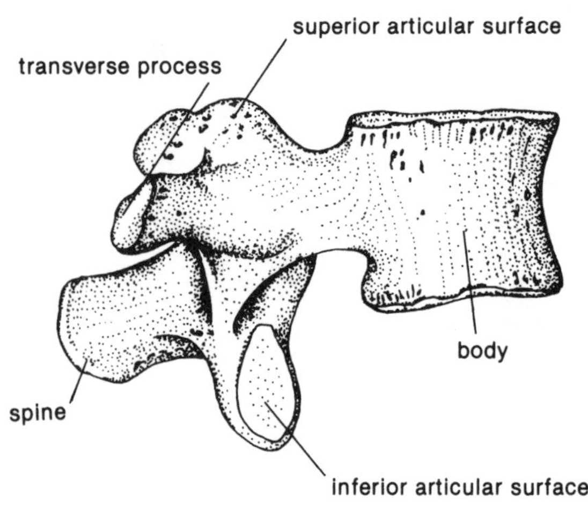

Figure 14: Lateral view of vertebra.

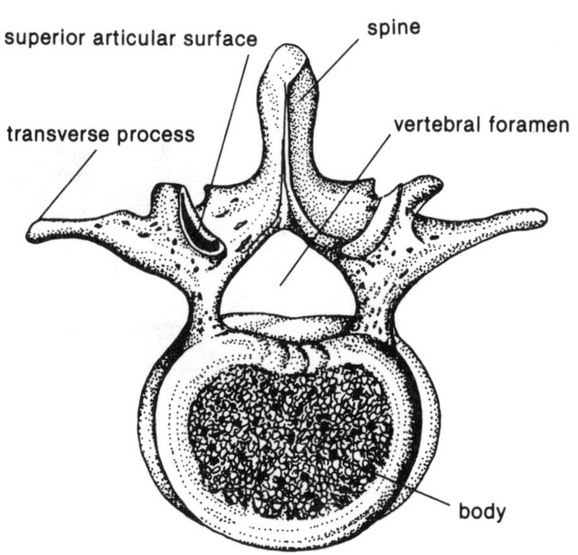

Figure 15: Superior view of vertebra.

outside of the back) forms the spine, which you can feel through the skin. The processes on the sides of the thoracic vertebrae are attached to the ribs. The inner process on all but the first two is called the **body**. It is the largest projection, and is filled with marrow.

The first and second **cervical vertebrae,** in the neck, are somewhat different from the rest, and have specific names (see Figure 16). The first is called the **atlas,** because it supports the head. The occipital bone of the cranium fits into two cup-like indentations on the surface of the atlas. These articular surfaces of the atlas. These articular surfaces allow the head to nod up and down. The second cervical vertebra is called the **axis.** It has a projection, called the **odontoid (oh DON toyd) process,** that fits neatly into the opening in the atlas between the transverse ligament and the spinal cord. This structure serves as a pivot, and allows the head to turn from side to side.

Occasionally, the transverse process of the seventh cervical vertebra forms a separate elongated bone called a cervical rib.

Each of the 12 thoracic vertebrae articulates with two ribs, one on either side of the body. The thoracic vertabrae gradually increase in size from top to bottom.

The lumbar vertebrae are distinguished by their large vertebral bodies, an appropriate characteristic since they support the weight of the entire upper body.

The sacrum, a large triangular bone, articulates with the fifth lumbar vertebra above, the coccyx below, and the pelvis (sacroiliac joint) on both sides. The five separate bones of the sacrum fuse between age 25 and 30 to form a single structure.

The coccyx, the lowest part of the spine, is formed of four fused bones. Fusion is usually completed by age 30.

The vertebral column (see Figure 17) is not perfectly straight when viewed from the side. It curves slightly slightly inward in the neck, outward in the chest, and inward again in the lower back. However, it is straight when viewed from the rear. In some people, because of disease and sometimes even because of poor posture, the curvature becomes distorted.

The condition called hunchback, technically known as **kyphosis (kye FOH sis),** occurs when the thoracic region of the spine curves too far outward. The slight inward curve of the cervical and lumbar regions is called **normal lordosis (lor DOH sis).** When it becomes excessive, the condition is called simply lordosis. The common terms for this are hollow back, saddle back, and swayback. The term **scoliosis (SKOH lee oh sis)** means abnormal vertical curvature, the spine is curved, instead of straight, when viewed from the rear. Scoliosis can occur in either sex, but is more common in women.

Thorax, or Chest Area. The bones of the thorax (see Figure 18 and Table 6) form a rounded, protective cage, narrower at the top than at the bottom, around the heart and lungs. Most of the ribs articulate with the body and the processes of the thoracic vertebrae in the back, and with the sternum in the front, thus making a complete circle around the chest.

The ribs (see Figure 19) curve outward from the vertebral column, then forward and

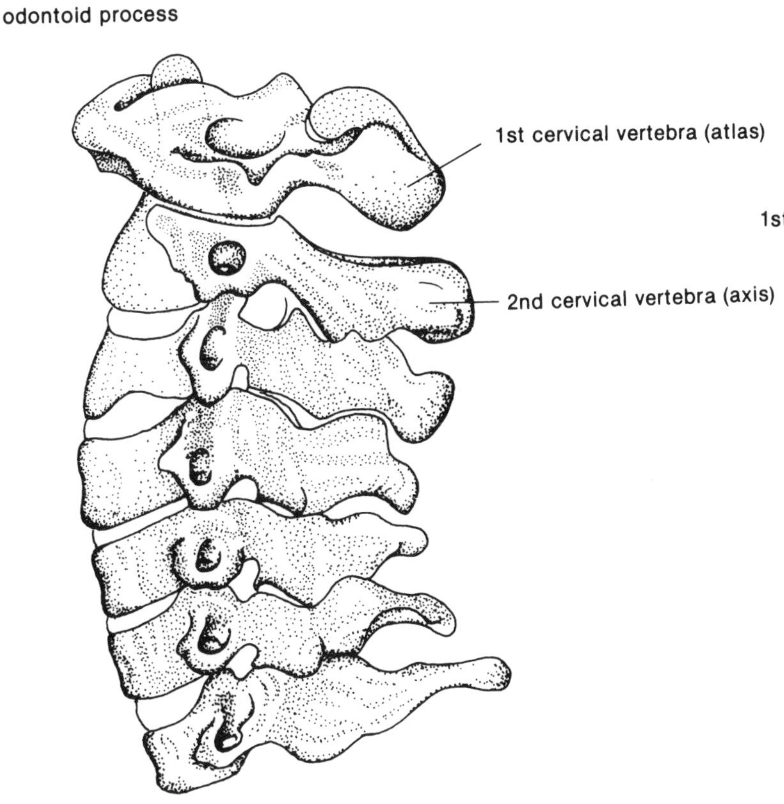

Figure 16: Lateral view of cervical spine.

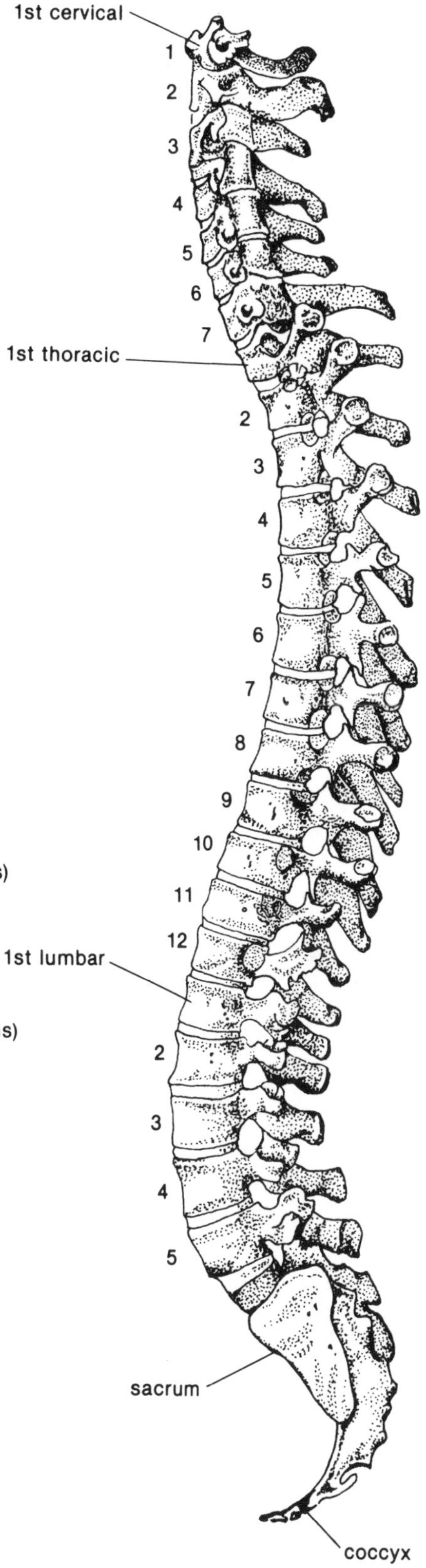

Figure 17: Lateral view of spinal column.

Table 6: The Bones of the Thorax, or Chest Area

Sternum breastbone	1
Ribs (costae)	
true (vertebrosternal) ribs	7 pairs
false ribs	5 pairs
vertebrochondral ribs	3 pairs
vertebral (floating) ribs	2 pairs

downward to the sternum. This shape, and the way the ribs are attached, allows them to move up and down as the lungs expand and contract during breathing.

The **sternum**, or breastbone (see Figure 20) is a long, flat bone that resembles a dagger blade. The heart normally lies beneath it and to the left. The sternum does not become completely ossified until well into adulthood, and the lowest part, called the **xiphoid (ZYE foyd) process** hardens last. There are muscles attached to this part, but the ribs are connected to the upper portions, the manubrium and the body of the sternum.

The ribs are also called the **costae (KOS tee)**. They are classified in two groups: the true ribs, which are attached to both the vertebrae and the sternum, and the false ribs, which are attached to the vertebrae but not to the sternum. There are seven pairs of true ribs, also called *vertebrosternal ribs*, and they are at the top of the ribcage. The five pairs of false ribs are divided again into two groups. The top three articulate with the ribs above them, and thus are indirectly attached to the sternum. The other two pairs are called *floating ribs*, because they are attached to the ver-

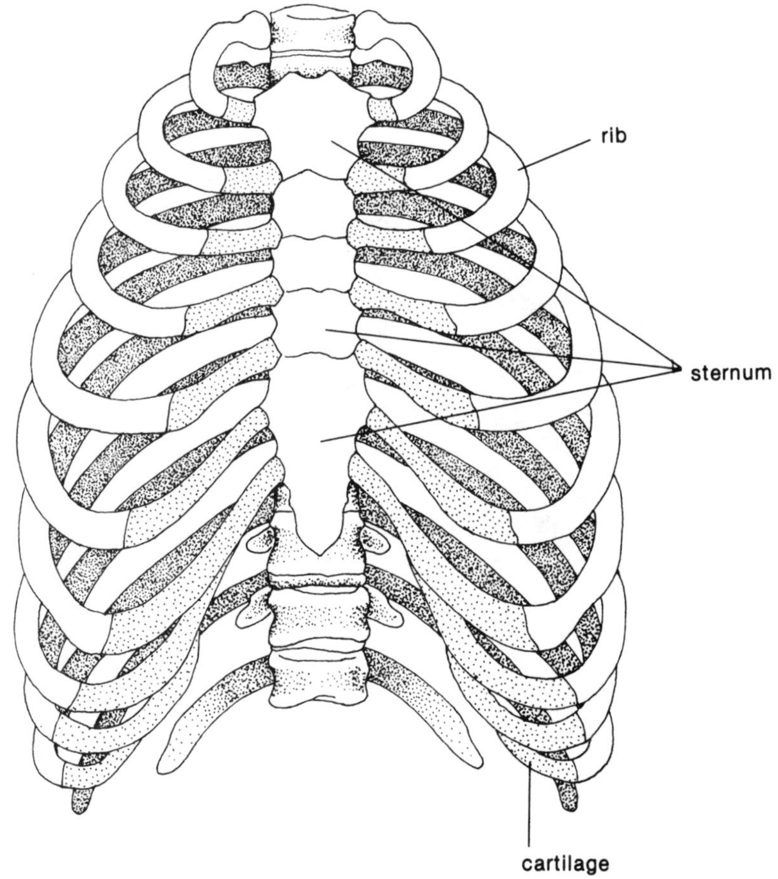

Figure 18: Anterior view of thoracic region.

tebrae in the back, but not in the front. The floating ribs are considerably shorter than the others.

The bones described above are all part of the axial, or central, skeleton. The remaining bones to be discussed are in the appendicular skeleton, or the limbs. (STOP AND RVIEW, page 26.)

Shoulder Bones. The shoulder bones form the shoulder girdle, which attaches the arms to the axial skeleton. Its four bones make an open circle, not a closed one like the ribs (see Table 7).

The **clavicles (KLAV ih kulz)** (see Figure 21) are slightly curved long bones located in the front of the body above the first pair of ribs. One end of each one articulates with the top of the sternum in the front, and the other end joins the scapula. The clavicles are the most frequently broken bones in the body.

Table 7: The Bones of the Shoulders

Clavicle	collar bone	2
Scapula	shoulder blade	2

Each **scapula (SKAP yuh lah)** (shoulder bone) is a flat, triangular-shaped bone with a prominent ridge on the back side (see Figures 22 and 23). The clavicles are joined to the scapulae at the outside end of this ridge, which is called the **acromion (ah KROH**

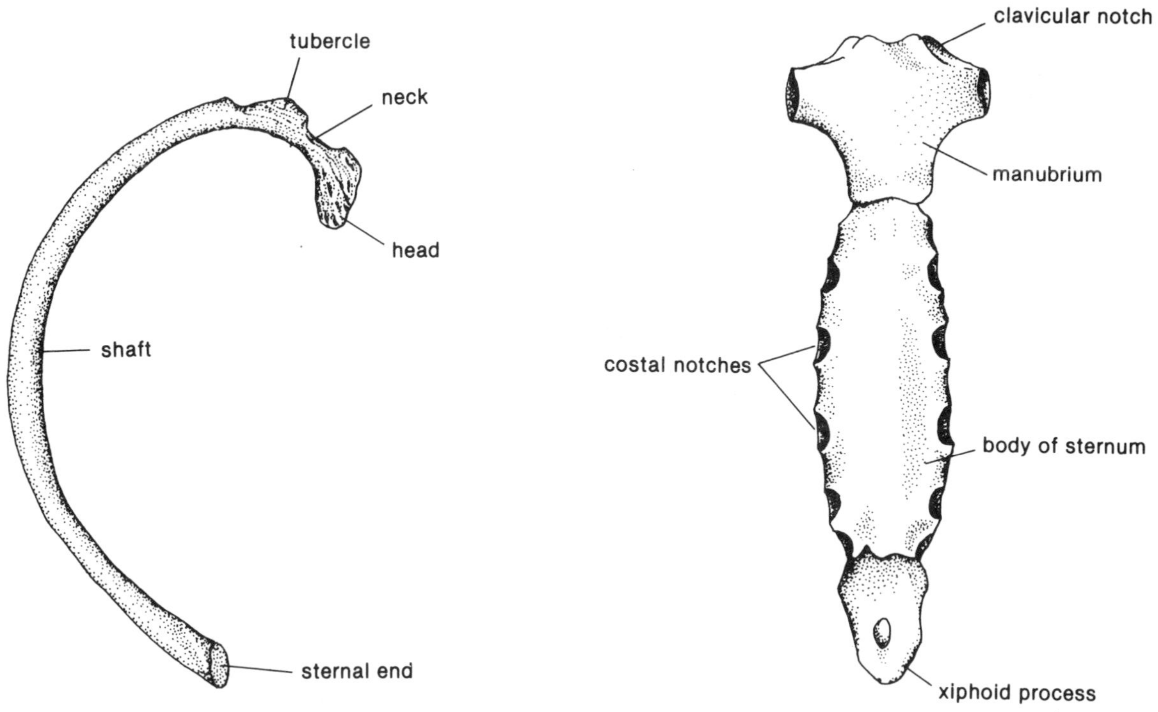

Figure 19: Superior view of rib.

Figure 20: Anterior view of sternum.

Figure 21: Anterior view of clavicle.

STOP AND REVIEW

1. Name two bones involved in chewing.

   a. ______________________

   b. ______________________

2. The chest organs are protected by which two bony structures?

   a. ______________________

   b. ______________________

3. Cavities within the facial and cranial bones are called ______________________ .

4. The slight inward curve of the cervical and lumbar regions of a normal spine is called ___ ______________________ .

5. The cartilage pads between the vertebrae are called ______________________ .

6. What results when the cartilage pads between the vertebrae slip out of position? _______ ______________________

True/False:

____7. Sinuses in the cranial and facial bones are part of the circulatory system.

____8. The axis (in the cervical spine) supports the head.

____9. The vertebrae contain marrow.

____10. Another name for the five pairs of vertebrochondral ribs is "true ribs."

11. Match these bones or parts of bones with their function.

a. atlas	____ 1. allows head to turn from side to side
b. axis	____ 2. allows head to nod up and down
c. odontoid process	____ 3. fits into the opening of the first vertebra
d. foramen magnum	____ 4. allows the spinal column to attach to the skull
	____ 5. contains marrow
	____ 6. attaches to the ribs

(continued next page)

mee on) process. The scapulae are located between the second and seventh ribs, across the back with the spine between them. They are attached to the ribs with muscles, not with joints. Just below the acromion process is another projection called the **glenoid fossa (GLEE noid FOS uh).** This is located roughly at the right angle of the triangle. Here the upper arm joins the shoulder and forms the shoulder joint (see Figure 6).

STOP AND REVIEW

12. Identify the labeled structures on the diagram below.

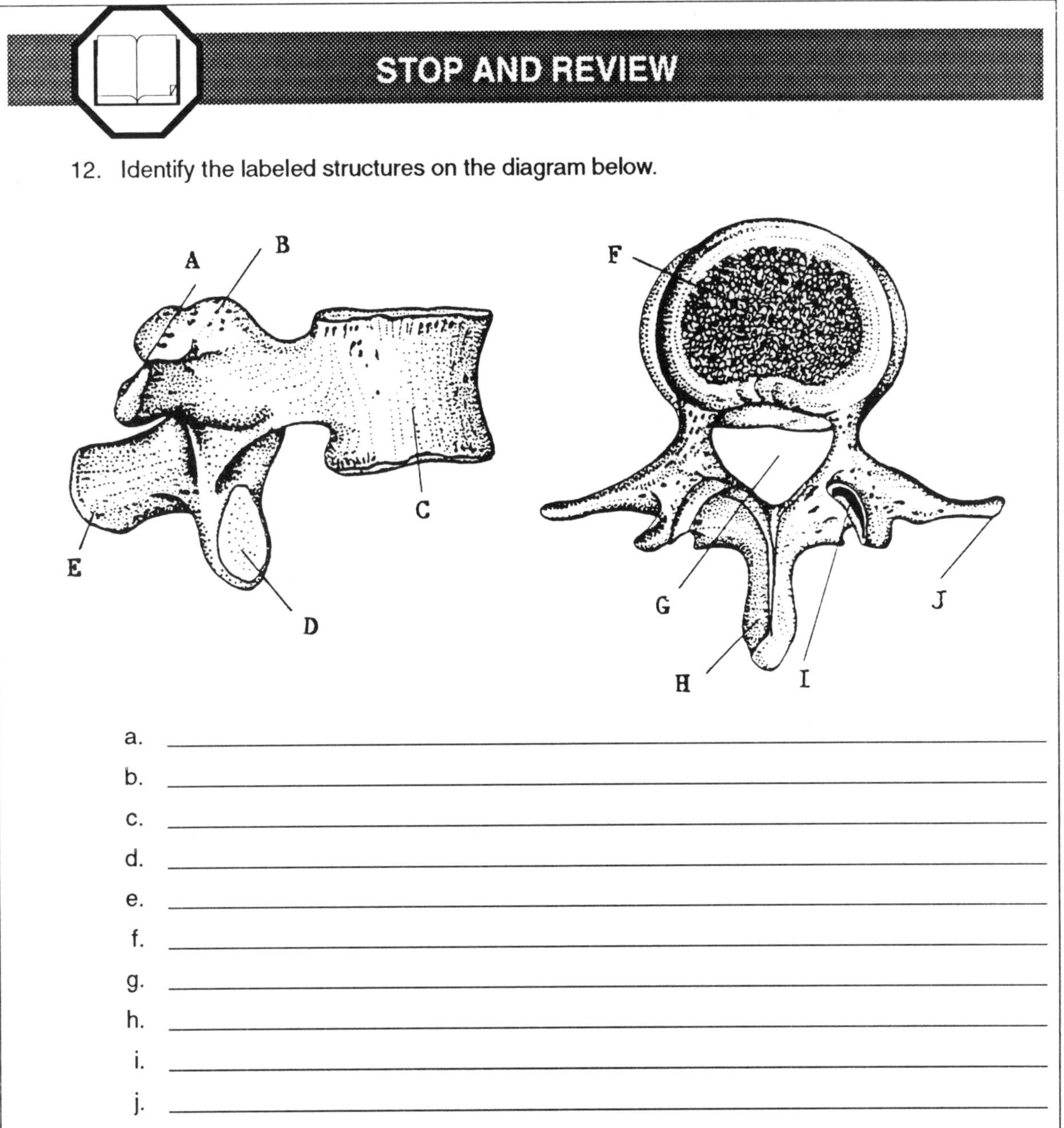

a. ______________________

b. ______________________

c. ______________________

d. ______________________

e. ______________________

f. ______________________

g. ______________________

h. ______________________

i. ______________________

j. ______________________

Arm, Wrist and Hand Bones. The upper extremities are made up of long bones in the arms, short bones in the wrists, and miniature long bones in the hands and fingers (see Table 8). The upper extremities are capable of very complex and precise movements, partly because of the number and design of the bones.

The **humerus (HYOOM er us)** (see Figures 24 and 25) is the upper arm bone, and is the longest and largest bone in the arm. Its upper end is rounded to fit into the glenoid fossa of the scapula and forms a ball-and-socket joint at the shoulder. At the lower end, the humerus has two rounded projections called the **capitulum (kah PIT yoo lum)** and the **trochlea (TROCK lee uh)**. These projections articulate with the bones of the forearm to form the elbow joint. The humerus also has a projection on the side called the **medial epicondyle (EP ih KON dyle)** which is sometimes referred to as the

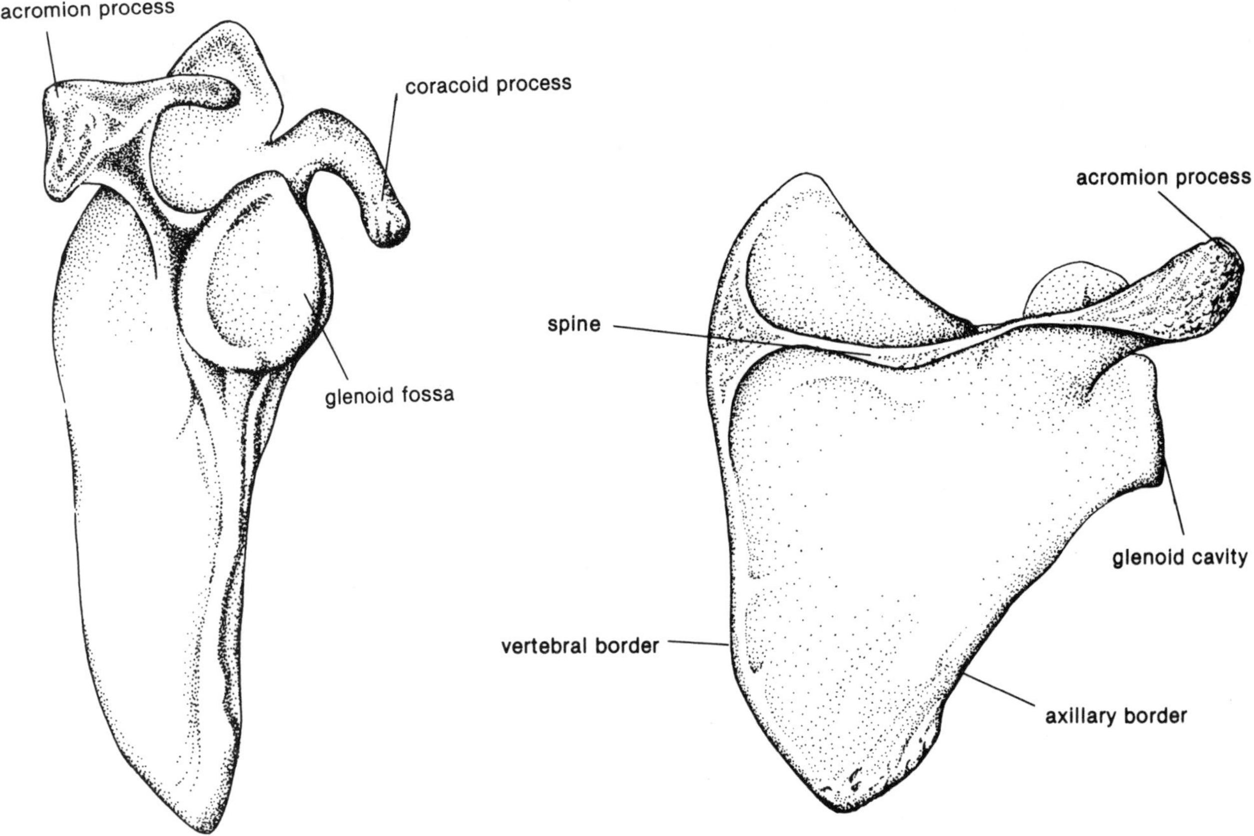

Figure 22: Lateral view of scapula.

Figure 23: Posterior view of scapula.

funny bone.

The **ulna** (see Figures 26 and 27) is the longer of the two forearm bones. At the top of it is a hook-shaped projection called the **olecranon (oh LECK ruh non)** which fits over the trochlea of the humerus at the elbow. At the wrist, the ulna does not articulate with the wrist bones. Instead, one side of it is separated from the wrist by a disk made of cartilage and fiber, and the other side is attached to the wrist by a ligament.

Table 8: Bones of the Arm, Wrist and Hand

Humerus	
upper arm	1 in each arm
Radius	
forearm, thumb side	1 in each arm
Ulna	
forearm, little finger side	1 in each arm
Carpals	
wrist bones	8 in each wrist
Metacarpals	
hand bones	5 in each hand
Phalanges	
finger bones	14 in each hand

The **radius** (see Figures 26 and 27) is both smaller and shorter than the ulna. It has a depression at its head that joins the humerus at the capitulum, and a ridge below the head that fits into a corresponding notch in the ulna. This structure allows the forearm to rotate at the elbow (see Figure 27). At the wrist, the radius articulates with the lunate and navicular bones of the wrist on one side and with the ulna on the other. Again, this structure allows the arm to rotate.

There are eight short bones in each wrist, called the **carpals (KAHR pulz)** (see Figure 28). They are arranged in two rows of four

BREAKS IN THE RADIUS AND ULNA

Only rarely is either the radius or ulna broken separately. Generally, trauma severe enough to break one bone will result in breaking both. Fractures of the distal radius and ulna are usually casted in a position midway between pronation (palm down) and supination (palm up). This is not only the most comfortable position, but it also increases spearation between the two bones, thus reducing the likelihood that they will fuse while healing.

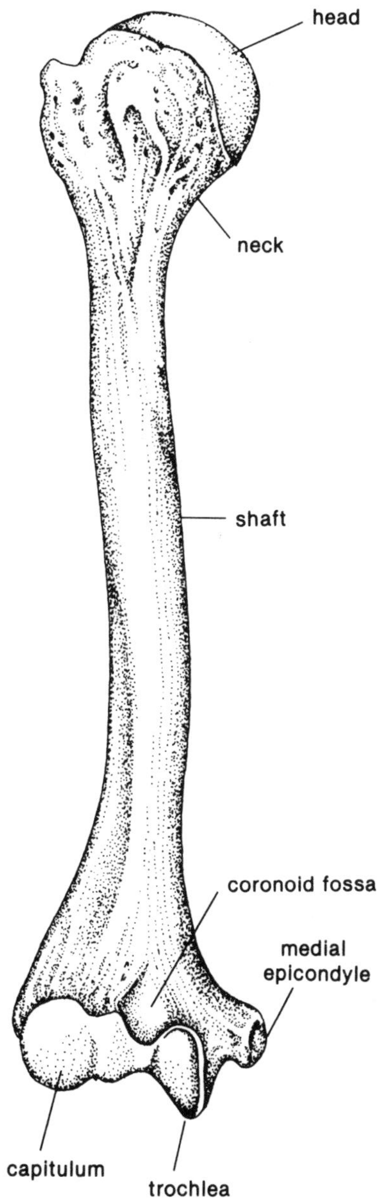

Figure 24: Anterior view of humerus.

each. In the proximal **(PROCK sih mul)** row (the row closest to the arm and body) are the **navicular (nah VICK yoo lur), lunate (LEW nayt), triangular (trye ANG gew lur),** and **pisiform (PYE sih form)** bones, moving from the thumb side to the little finger side. The distal row, or the row closest to the hand and most distant from the body, includes the **greater** and **lesser multangular (mul TANG gew lur),** the **capitate (KAP ih tate),** and the **hamate (HAY mate)** bones, again from thumb to little finger. These bones are joined together with ligaments, so that they are held in place but are able to move to some extent.

The bones of the hand are called **metacarpals (MET uh KARH pulz).** There are five of them, and they are identified by number. The first metacarpal is the one on the thumb side. The metacarpals articulate with the wrist bones (carpals) at one end and with the fingers at the other end. The knuckles mark the point where the metacarpals articulate with the finger bones. The first metacarpal is the most frequently broken hand bone, followed by the second, fourth, and fifth metacarpals.

The finger bones are called **phalanges (fa LAN jeez)** (phalanx, singular); this term is also used for the bones of the toes. There are 14 phalanges in each hand, three in each finger, and two in the thumb. In the thumb they are called *proximal* (close to the body) and *distal* (far from the body) phalanges, and in each finger they are the proximal, middle, and distal phalanges.

Pelvic Girdle. The **pelvic girdle** (see Figures 29 and 30) supports the legs and thus the whole body when standing. It also protects

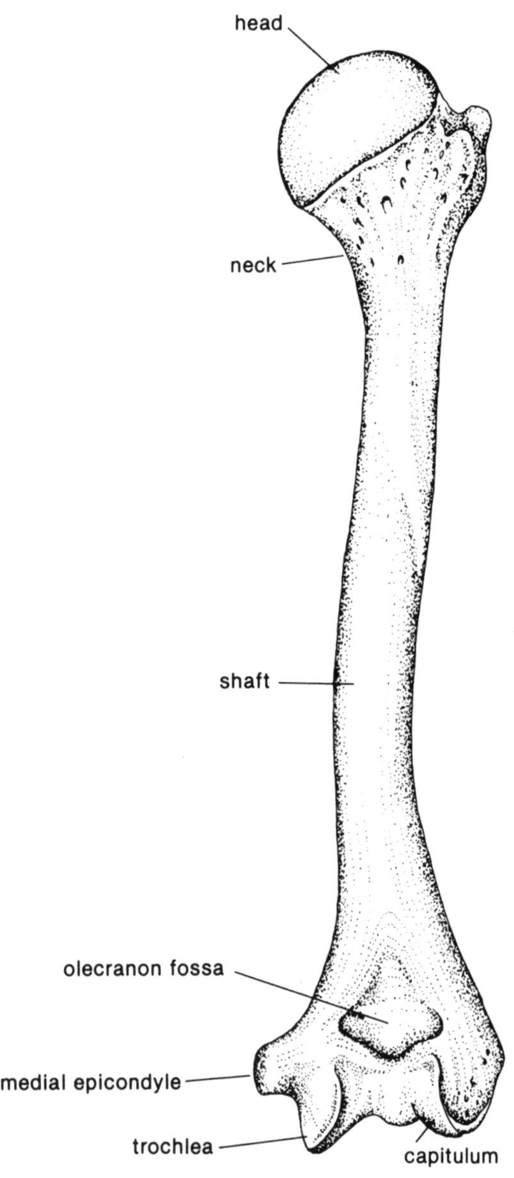

Figure 25: Posterior view of humerus.

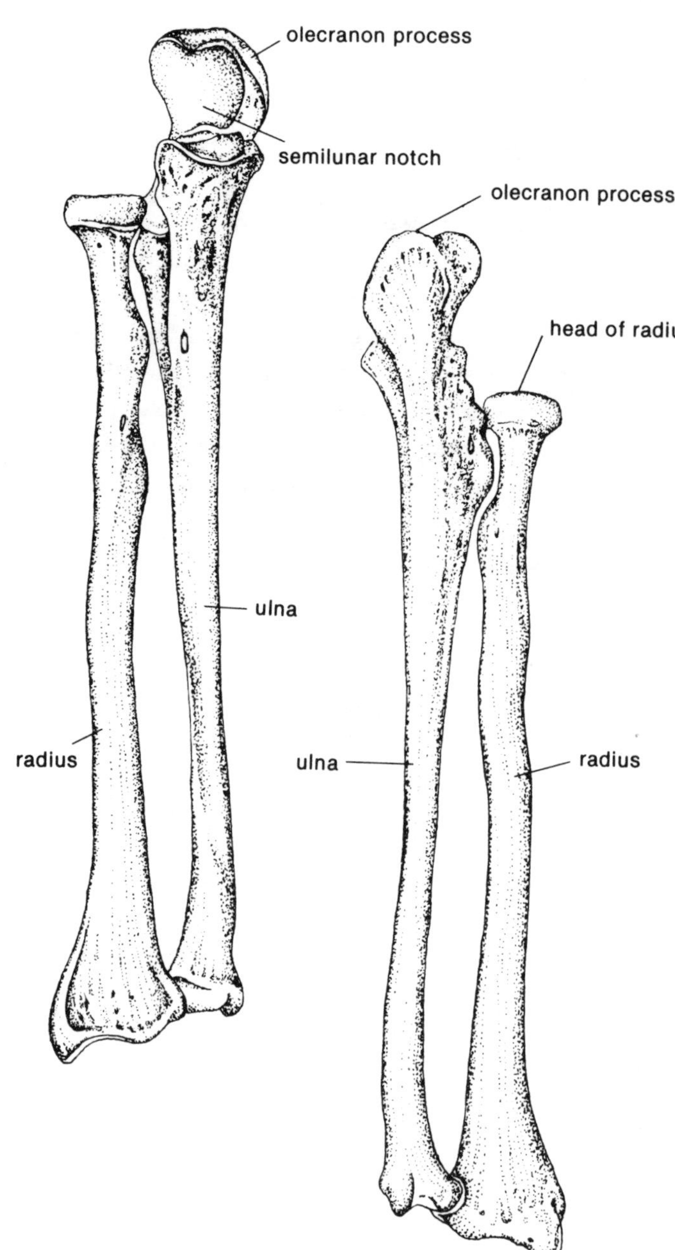

Figure 26: Anterior and posterior views of lower arm, showing rotation.

part of the intestines, the bladder, and the reproductive organs in women. The pelvic bones are connected to each other in the front and to the sacrum and coccyx (parts of the vertebral column) in the back. Together they form a circular framework, with a large opening in the middle, that surrounds the organs.

Each of the two matching pelvic bones is made up of three separate bones at birth. These bones gradually unite, but the names of the original parts are still used for the corresponding regions of the pelvic bone. The upper portion, which juts out to form the hip, is called the **ilium (IL ee um).** The curved edge of the ilium is called the *iliac crest*. The lowest portion, which forms a loop below the front of the pelvis, is called the **ischium (IS kee um).** The third part, which is in front and closes the circle by meeting the corresponding part of the opposite hip bone, is called the **pubis**. The ilium joins the sacrum at a joint called the **sacroiliac (SACK**

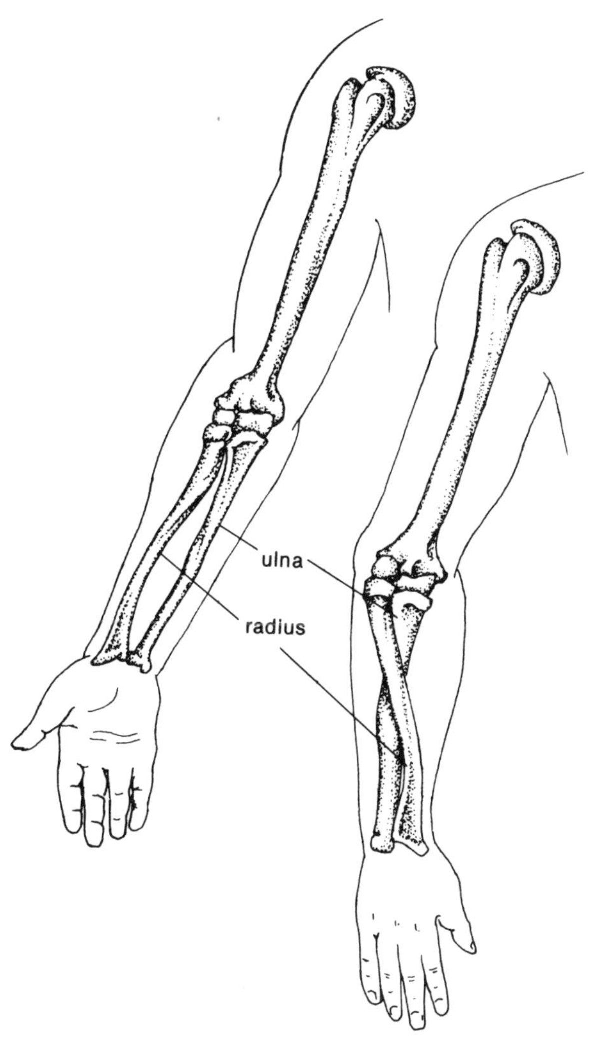

Figure 27: Anterior view of the lower arm, showing rotation.

roh IL ee ack) joint. The socket for the hip joint is found at the point where the three parts of the hip bone come together. It is called the **acetabulum (AS eh TAB yoo lum).**

The male and female pelvises (see Figure 30) have slightly different shapes. The female pelvis must be wide enough to allow a full-term baby to be delivered through the central opening. Therefore, the female pelvis is wider and flatter than the male pelvis, and the female coccyx is more flexible.

Leg, Ankle, and Foot Bones. The legs, or lower extremities, must be strong enough to support and move the whole body (see Table 9). They are therefore sturdier in structure and heavier than the bones of the arms. The legs are also less movable than the arms.

The **femur (FEE mur)** (see Figure 31) is the heaviest bone in the human skeleton. The head of the femur joins the pelvic bone at the acetabulum, forming a ball-and-socket joint similar to the one at the shoulder. Just below the head are two bulges in the bone called the **greater** and **lesser trochanters (tro KAN turz).** At the other end, at the knee joint, are two rounded bulges in the bone called the **medial condyle (MEE dee ul KON dyle)** and the **lateral condyle (LAT ur ul KON dyle).** These join with corresponding condyles on the tibia.

The **patella (pah TELL uh),** or kneecap (see Figure 32), is the only named sesamoid bone in the body, mainly because it is the largest. **Sesamoid (SES uh moid) bones** are usually about the size and shape of a sesame seed, which are formed in the tendons. The patella lies in front of the knee joint to protect it and improve the leverage of the leg muscles. The patella may be fractured by falls directly on the knee, or by a strong muscular contraction such as might be encountered in athletic activities.

The **tibia (TIB ee uh)** is the shinbone, the bone at the front of the lower leg (see Figure 33). It is larger and stronger than the fibula, and is called the **medial** bone of the leg because it is located in the center, or median. At the lower end of the tibia is a process or projection, called the **medial malleolus**

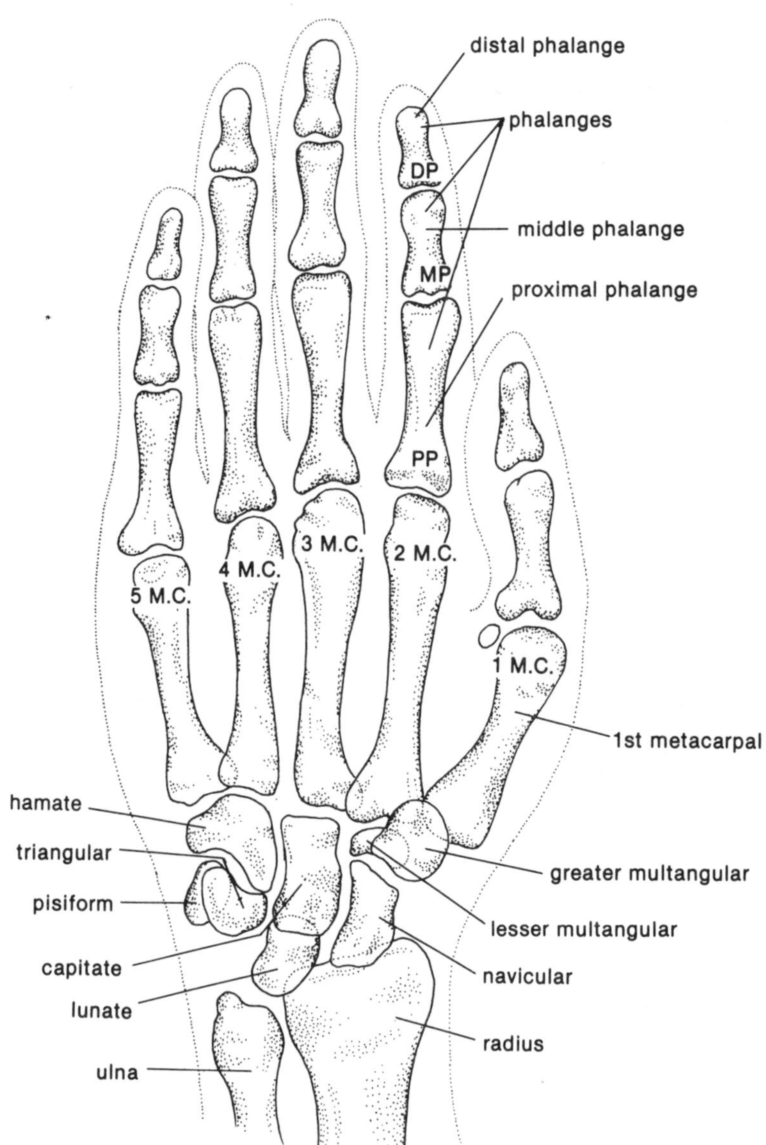

Figure 28: Posterior view of left hand.

(mah LEE oh lus), which forms part of the ankle joint.

The **fibula (FIB yuh luh)** is placed parallel to the tibia. It does not join the femur at the knee. Instead, it articulates with the tibia below the joint. At the other end of this slender bone is a process called the **lateral malleolus**, which forms the ankle joint with the medial malleolus of the tibia and the talus, one of

FRACTURES OF THE FEMUR

A broken hip is actually a fracture of the femur. Fractures of the femoral neck are common in elderly people, particularly among women. This may be caused by degenerative changes due to poor nutrition or physical inactivity. Femoral fractures through the greater and lesser trochanters are usually caused by falls or other injuries. In both cases, surgical implantation of steel rods or artificial hip joints is frequently required to correct the problem.

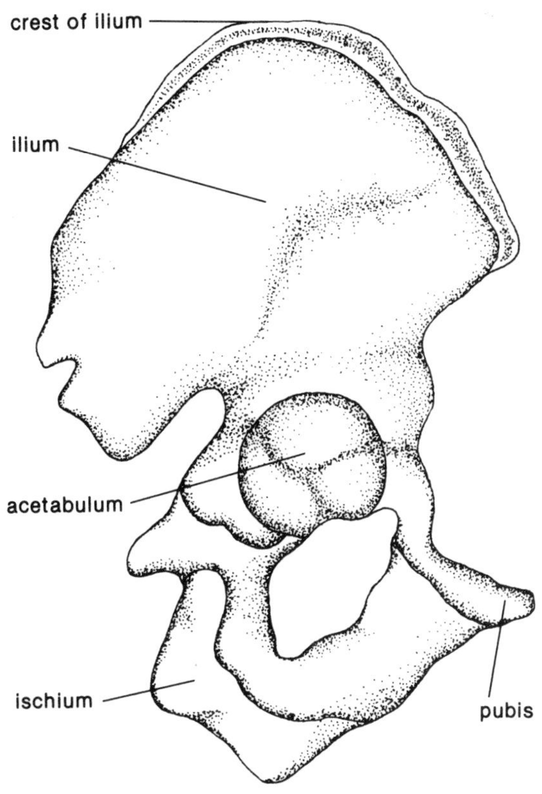

Figure 29: Lateral view of pelvis.

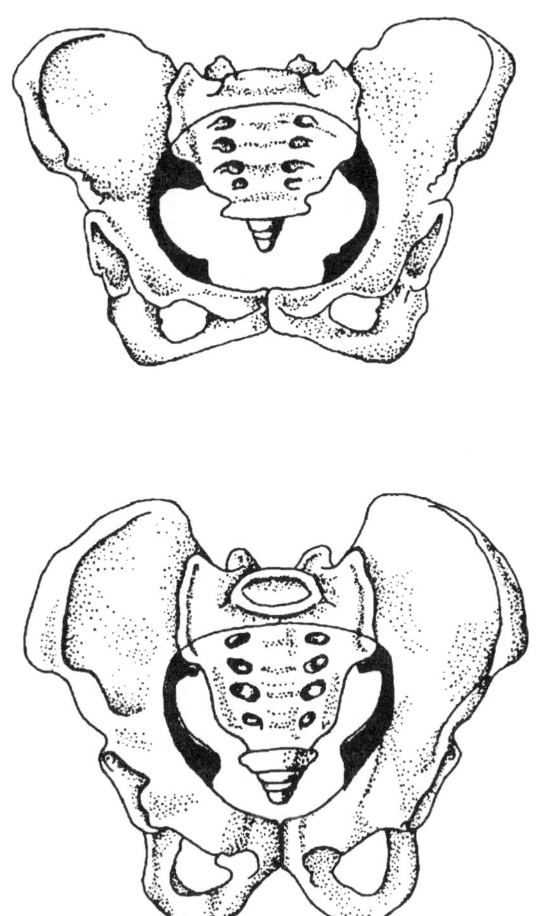

Figure 30: Anterior views of female (top) and male (bottom) pelvises.

Table 9: Bones of the Leg, Ankle, and Foot

Femur	
thigh bone	1 in each leg
Patella	
kneecap	1 in each leg
Tibia	
shinbone	1 in each leg
Fibula	
calf bone	1 in each leg
Tarsals	
ankle bones	7 in each ankle
Metatarsals	
foot bones	5 in each foot
Phalanges	
toes	14 in each foot

the ankle bones.

The seven **tarsals (TAHR sulz)** are the **talus (TAY lus)** which forms a joint with the lower leg bones; the **calcaneus (kal KAY nee us)** or heel; the **navicular (nah VICK yoo lur)**; the **cuboid (KEW boyd)**; and the three **cuneiforms (kew NEE ih formz).** The cuneiforms (on the inside edge) and cuboid (on the outside edge) are closest to the metatarsals, and the navicular is in the center of the foot on the inside edge (see Figures 34 and 35).

The five metatarsals are numbered from the inside edge of the foot to the outside edge. They are long bones, like the metacarpals of the hands. The phalanges, like the finger bones, are miniature long bones. They are arranged in the same way, with two in

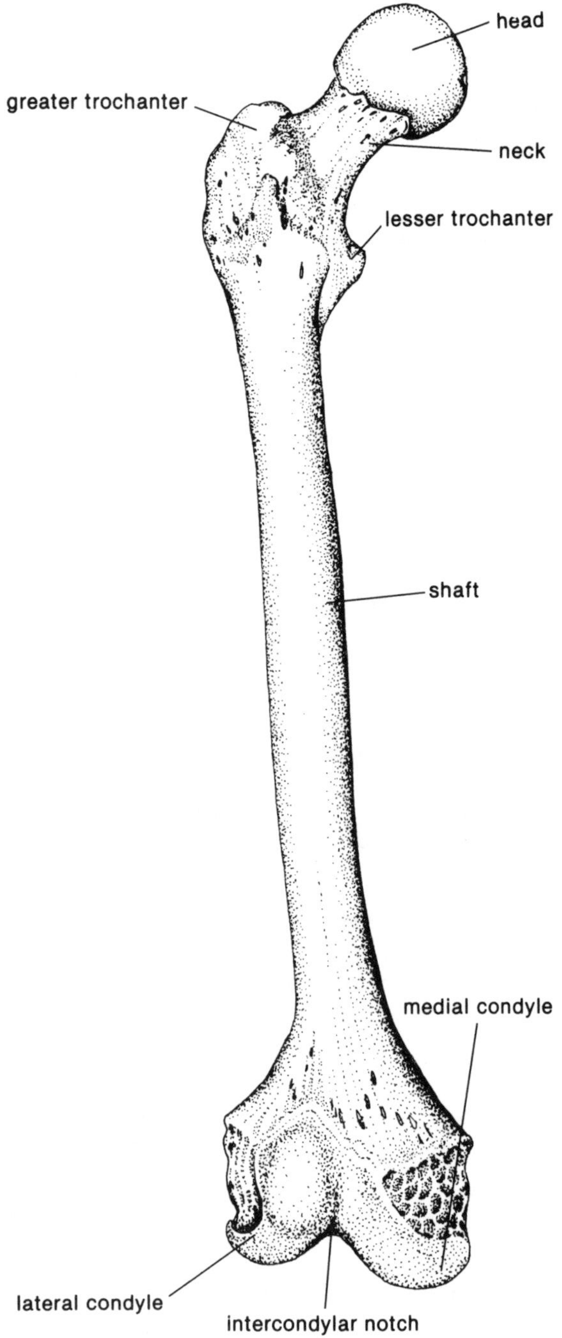

Figure 31: Anterior view of right femur.

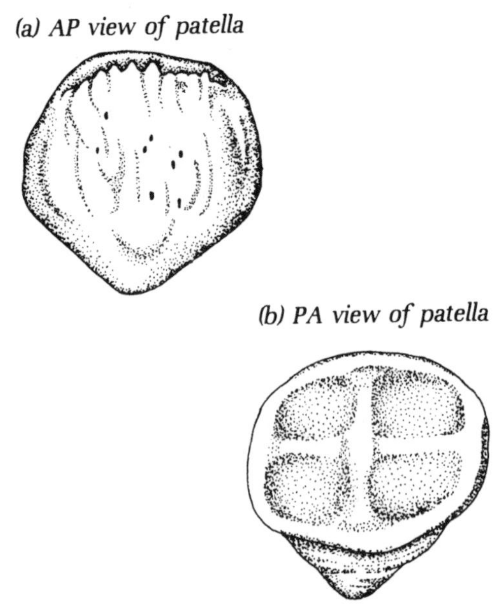

Figure 32: Anterior-posterior (AP) and posterior-anterior (PA) views of patella.

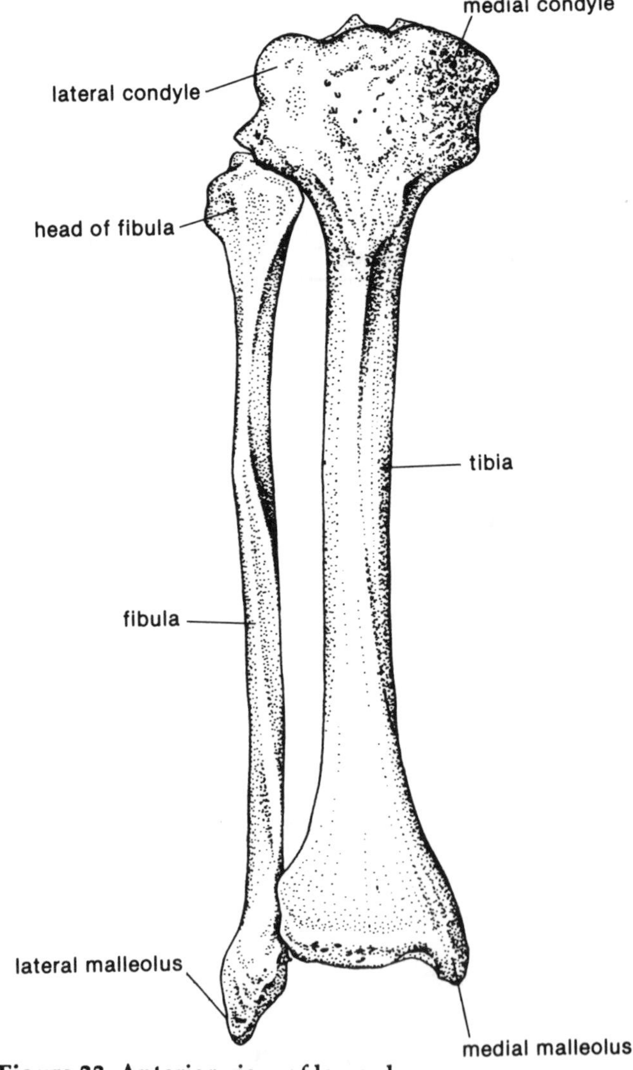

Figure 33: Anterior view of lower leg.

the big toes and three in each of the other toes.

The feet are heavier than the hands, and their bones are larger, because of the weight the feet must support. Also, the foot is shaped into two arches, which is the strongest possible type of construction (see Figure 36). One of the arches stretches from the heel to the toes, and is called the **longitudinal arch**. The other is from side to side, and is called the **transverse arch**. Both arches are held in place by the muscles and tendons of the foot. (STOP AND REVIEW, page 36.)

ARTICULATIONS

The term articulation means junction or union between two bones of the skeleton. There are two types of articulation: **synar-**

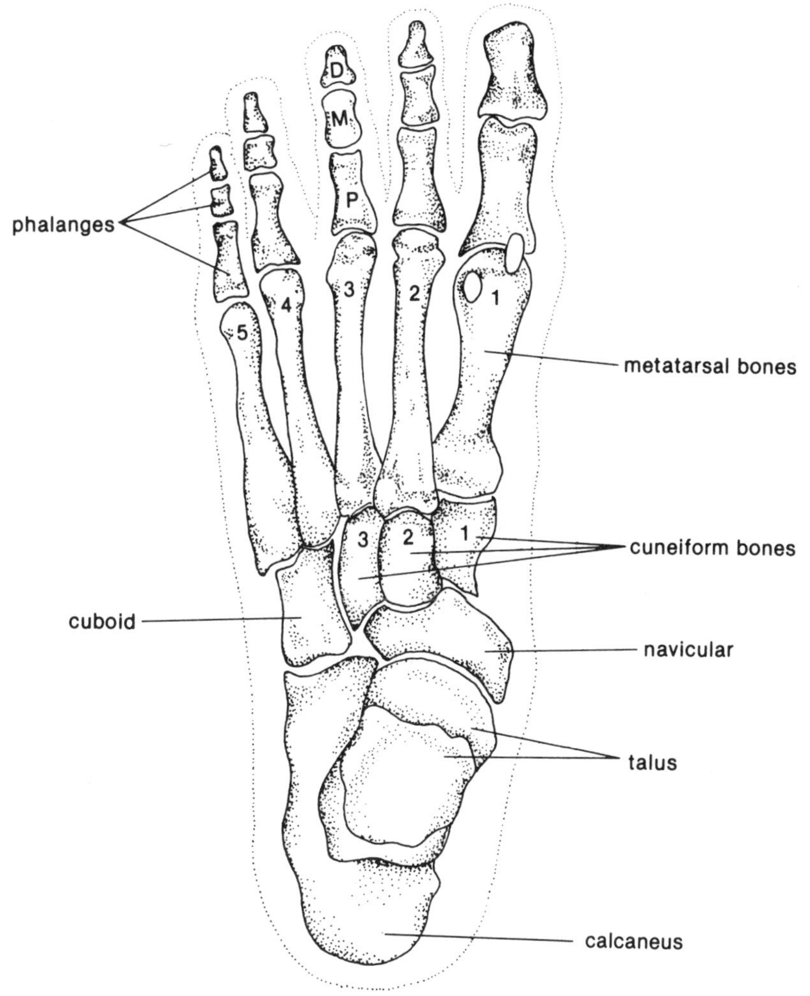

Figure 34: Superior view of foot.

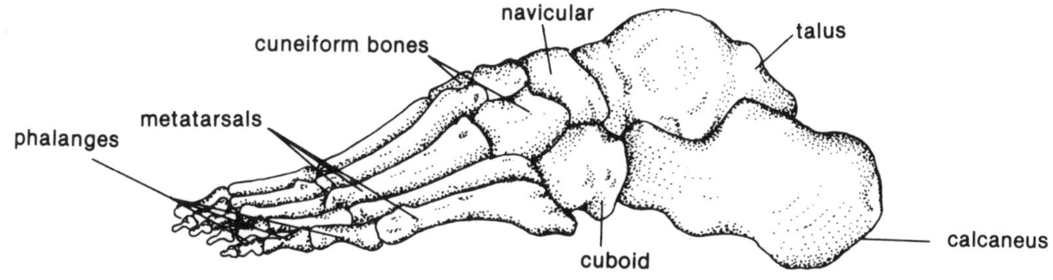

Figure 35: Lateral view of foot.

STOP AND REVIEW

Fill in the blanks for questions 1 through 4.

1. The ______________________________ is attached with muscles rather than joints.
   a. clavicle
   b. glenoid fossa
   c. scapula
2. The shoulder girdle attaches the arms to the ______________________ skeleton.
3. The bones of the hand are ______________________________ in shape.
4. The knuckles mark the point where the __________________ articulate with the ____.

Circle the correct answer.

5. The ulna and the radius comprise the:
   a. upper arm
   b. lower arm
6. The longest bone in the arm is the:
   a. radius
   b. olecranon
   c. carpal
   d. humerus
7. Place a *P* beside the names of the bones in the wrist that are closest to the body (proximal). Place a *D* beside the names of the bones in the wrist that are farthest from the body (distal).

______ olecranon	______ulna
______capitate	______lunate
______ navicular	______hamate
______ triangular	______lesser multangular
______ greater multangular	______pisiform
______ metacarpal	______phalanx

8. Check the bones or parts of bones that comprise the elbow joint.

______ phalanx	______ radius
______ ulna	______ tibia
______ medial epicondyle	______ trochlea
______ olecranon	______ metacarpal
______ capitulum	______ humerus

throses (SYN ahr THROH seez), in which the bones are held rigidly together, and **diarthroses (DYE ahr THROW seez),** in which there is a joint structure to allow movement.

In a synarthrosis, the space between the bones is filled with cartilage and fibrous connective tissue. In some cases the union of the bones permits almost no movement. An example of this is the sutures that hold together the bones of the cranium. In other cases, the bones are able to move slightly, to give with movements of the body. These unions are sometimes called **amphiarthroses (AM fee ahr THROW seez).** Some examples are the joints between the vertebrae, the sacroiliac joint in the pelvic girdle, and the joint between the tibia and fibula at the ankle.

Most of the articulations in the body are diarthroses, which are also called **synovial (sye NO vee al) joints.** Their structure is complex and has several elements (see Figure 37). Each one is surrounded by a fibrous joint capsule, which is an extension of the periosteum of each of the two bones. Within this capsule is a space between the bones. It is filled with synovial fluid and lined with a moist, slippery synovial membrane. **Bursae (BUR see),** or sacs, are made of membrane

CLUBFOOT

Clubfoot (talipes) is a deformity of the tarsal bones that causes the foot to be twisted out of its normal position. There are several types of clubfoot. Treatment consists of using casts and braces to correct the foot's alignment, or, in severe cases, even surgery.

DIARTHROTIC JOINT EXAMINATION

Diarthrotic joints can be examined using an x-ray procedure called arthrography. A radiopaque contrast medium is injected into the joint capsule and a series of radiographs is taken to detect injury or disease of the joint capsule. Arthrography outlines some tissues not typically seen on standard radiographs, such as knee cartilage and ligaments, as well as structures of the joint capsule.

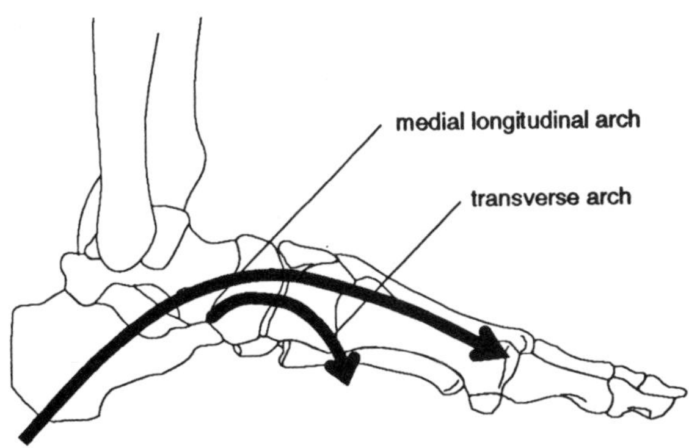

Figure 36: Transverse and longitudinal arches of the foot.

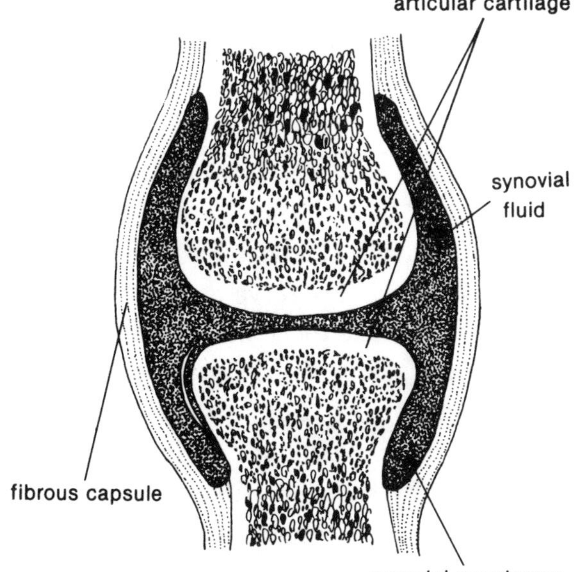

Figure 37: Synovial joint.

STOP AND REVIEW

Fill in the blanks for questions 1 through 5.

1. Two functions of the pelvic girdle are to

   a. ______________________________

   b. ______________________________

2. Each pelvic bone is composed of ______________ separate bones at birth.
3. The long bones in the foot are called ______________________.
4. The feet are shaped into two arches, the ______________________ arch from heel to toes and the ______________________ arch from side to side.
5. The sacroiliac joint has that name because it is the point where the ______________ joins the ______________________.

Circle the correct answers to questions 6 and 7.

6. The leg bone that joins the pelvic bone at the acetabulum is the

   a. patella

   b. tibia

   c. talus

   d. femur

7. The coccyx is more flexible in the

   a. male

   b. female

8. True/False: The sacrum, coccyx, pubis, and iliac crest are all parts of the pelvic girdle.

(continued next page)

and filled with synovial fluid, are also inside the capsule. They serve as cushions for the moving parts of the joint. The bones are held together inside the capsule by **ligaments,** which are strong, dense, fibrous cords. Thus the bones are held together on the outside of the joint by the sleeve-like capsule, and on the inside by ligaments, but the space between the bones remains open so that the bones can move freely. The **tendons** are similar to the ligaments but are larger and longer. They attach the muscles to the bones. The muscles then provide the power to move the joints.

Depending on how the bones are shaped and how the ligaments are arranged, the joint may be able to move in a number of different ways. For a list of different types of synovial joints, see Table 10 and Figure 38.

STOP AND REVIEW

9. Identify the labeled structures on the diagrams below.

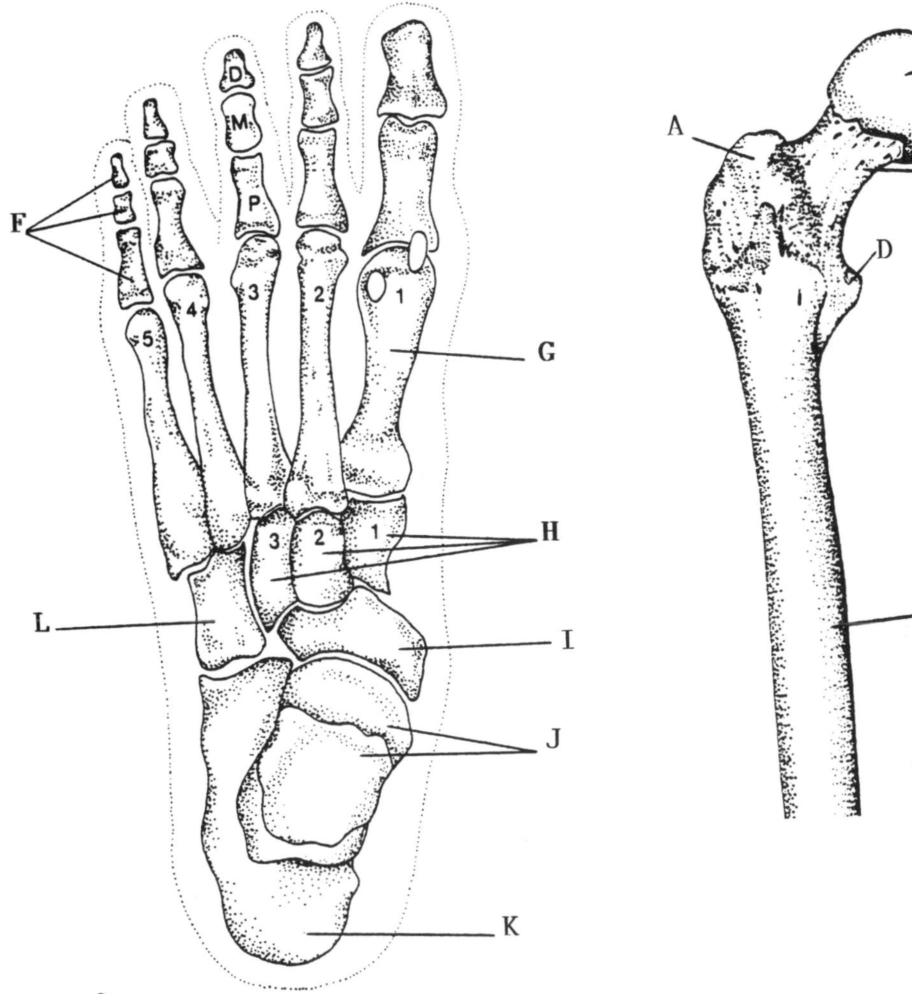

a. ______

b. ______

c. ______

d. ______

e. ______

f. ______

g. ______

h. ______

i. ______

j. ______

k. ______

l. ______

Table 10: Types of Synovial Joints

Joint Name	Example	Movements
Saddle	Thumb at wrist	Flexion, extension, abduction, adduction, circumduction
Hinge	Elbow, between humerus and lower arm	Flexion, extension
Pivot	Elbow, between radius and ulna	Rotation
Ellipsoidal	Wrist to arm	Flexion, extension, abduction, adduction
Gliding	Within wrist	Simple motion only
Ball-and-socket	Hip, shoulder	Flexion, extension, abduction, adduction, rotation, circumduction

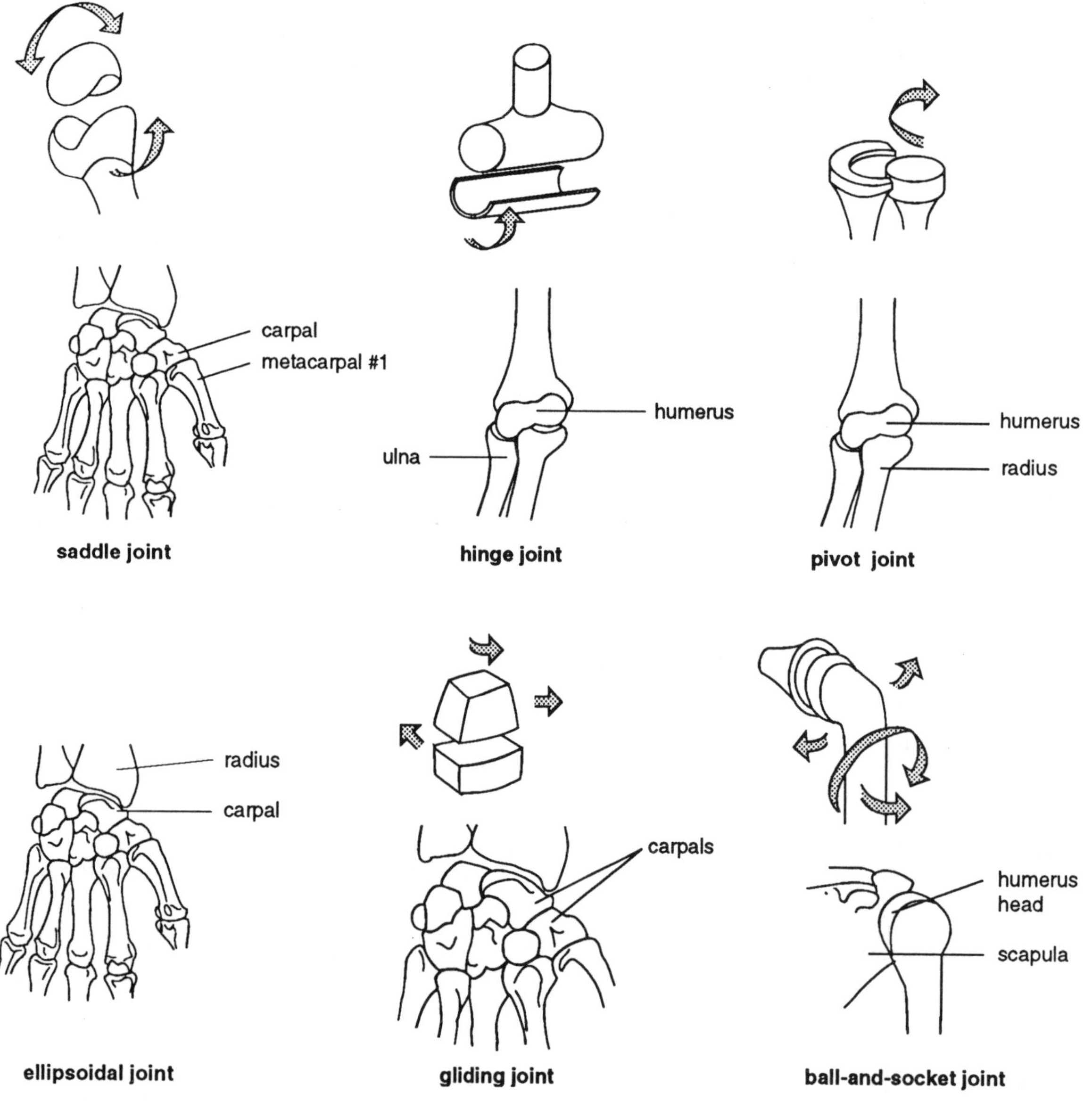

Figure 38: Types of sinovial joints.

STOP AND REVIEW

Fill in the blanks for questions 1 through 5.

1. A junction or union between two bones in the skeleton is called a(n) ________________ .
2. Space between bones, filled with cartilage and fibrous connective tissue, is a joint that allows ____ movement.
3. Bones in a diarthrotic joint are held together on the inside by ________________ .
4. Joints in the human body allow ________________ different kinds of movement.
5. A joint capsule is an extension of the
   a. medullary cavity
   b. synovial joint
   c. bursae
   d. periosteum
6. True/False: Ligaments attach muscles to bones.
7. Match each word with the correct definition:

a. synarthrosis	____1. bones held rigidly together
b. diarthrosis	____2. slight movement possible
c. amphiarthrosis	____3. joint that allows movement
	____4. joint allowing complete rotation

8. Match each type of joint with an example:

a. saddle	____1. neck
b. hinge	____2. elbow
c. pivot	____3. jaw
d. ellipsoidal	____4. shoulder
e. gliding	____5. within wrist
f. ball-and-socket	____6. knee
	____7. hip
	____8. wrist to arm
	____9. thumb at wrist

(continued next page)

Types of Body Movement

The joints allow 13 different kinds of movement.

1. **Flexion** is bending, or movement, forward from an the anatomical (rest) position.

STOP AND REVIEW

9. Match each movement with the action it allows:

a. circumduction	____ 1.	turning the head
b. protraction	____ 2.	turning the sole inward
c. rotation	____ 3.	winding up for a pitch
d. hyperextension	____ 4.	tilting the head backward
e. adduction	____ 5.	sticking out the tongue
f. abduction	____ 6.	moving a limb away from the center of the body
	____ 7.	moving a limb back toward the center of the body

2. **Extension** is returning from flexion to the anatomical position. It is the opposite of flexion.
3. **Hyperextension** is bending backward. An example is tilting the head back to look up.
4. **Adduction** is lateral, or sideways, movement away from the midline or center. An example is lifting the arm away from the body.
5. **Adduction** is returning from abduction to the midline.
6. **Circumduction** is circular movement, as in winding up to pitch a ball.
7. **Rotation** is pivoting movement, without moving from the central point. An example is rotating the head on the neck.
8. **Supination** is turning the palms upward or forward.
9. **Pronation** is turning the palms downward or backward.
10. **Inversion** is turning the sole inward.
11. **Eversion** is turning the sole outward.
12. **Protraction** is lowering the jaw or sticking out the tongue.
13. **Retraction** is raising the jaw or pulling the tongue back.

See Table 10 for information on which joints can make which movements. None of the joints can rotate completely, because such movement would tear the tissues that hold the joints together. (STOP AND REVIEW, page 41.)

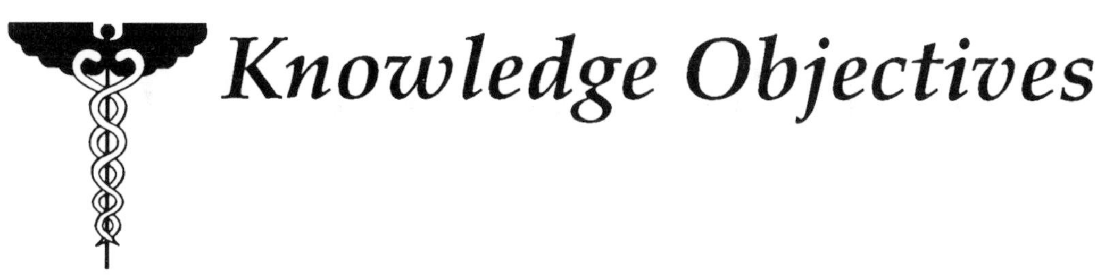

Knowledge Objectives

After completing this chapter, you should be able to:

Muscular System Function

- describe three kinds of muscle
- describe three major functions of muscle
- describe the location and function of endomysium, perimysium, and epimysium
- describe the structure of a muscle cell

Muscle Contraction

- describe the mechanism of muscle contraction
- describe the energy source for muscle contraction
- describe two major types of muscle contraction responsible for most body movement
- define *twitch, summation,* and *tetanus*

Specific Muscles

- locate and name the muscles of the:
    - face, head, and neck
    - shoulders, arms, hands, and wrists
    - abdomen
    - hips and legs
- describe how the respiratory muscles function

CHAPTER 2

The Muscular System

FUNCTIONS OF THE MUSCULAR SYSTEM

The bones and the joints are not of much use if there is no mechanism for moving them. The muscles and the associated nerves, tendons, and connective tissue provide that mechanism. There are three kinds of muscles. Of the three, only the skeletal muscles will be discussed in detail here (see Figure 39). **Skeletal muscles** are **striated (STRYE ay tid)** voluntary muscles. Striated means they appear to exhibit striations or bands when seen through a microscope. Voluntary means they are moved by conscious decisions.

The second kind of muscle is **cardiac,** or heart, **muscle** which is involuntary (not consciously controlled) and striated. The third kind is **visceral (VIS ur ul) muscle,** which is nonstriated (smooth) and involuntary. Visceral muscle controls the automatic activities of the body, such as digestion and breathing.

The skeletal muscles are the "meat" of the body. They account for between 40 percent and 50 percent of body weight. Skeletal muscles have three major functions, the first of which is movement, or contraction. The other functions of this kind of muscle are to generate body heat by their activity, and maintain body posture when a person is sitting or standing. This third function can be illustrated by the fact that a person who loses consciousness falls down or slumps over. The voluntary muscles do not contract unless they are stimulated. When someone loses consciousness, stimulation of the skeletal muscles stops, and the function of maintaining posture ceases.

Like bones, muscles are not the simple structures that they appear to be to the unassisted eye. Each named muscle is made up of many muscle cells, and covered with connective tissue (see Figure 40). Each individual cell, also called a **muscle fiber,** is wrapped in a covering called an **endomysium (EN doh MIS ee um).** Groups of cells within the muscle are wrapped with a **perimysium (PERR ih MIS ee um).**

Finally, the entire structure is covered by an **epimysium (EP ih MIS ee um).** In addition to providing protection for the muscle, these wrappings combine with the tendons to hold the muscles in place on the skeleton. The tendons are strong, flexible, cord-like tissues that are continuous with the epimysium on the outside of the muscle and the periosteum on the outside of the bone.

Structure of a Muscle Cell

Each muscle cell is long and thin and has many **nuclei (NOO klee eye)** (see Figure 41). The outer membrane of the cell is called

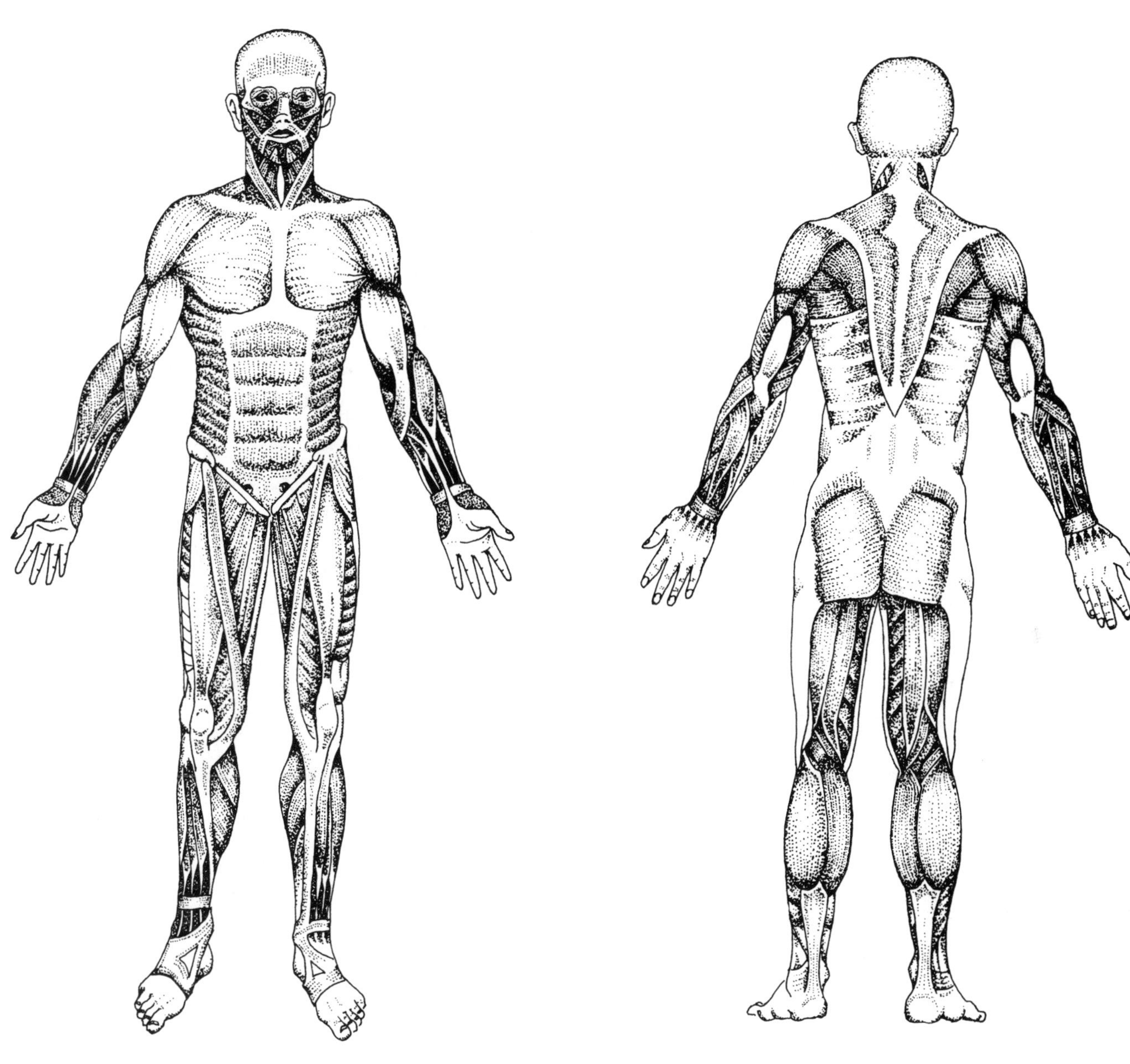

Figure 39: Anterior and posterior views of skeletal muscles.

the **sarcolemma (SAHR koh LEM uh).** It contains the **sarcoplasm (SAHR koh PLAZ um)** or main body of the cell, and the nuclei. Within the sarcoplasm are three major structures: the **sarcoplasmic reticulum (SAHR koh PLAZ mick re TICK yoo lum)** is a network of canals with tiny sacs at the ends that contain calcium. These canals run parallel to the fibers themselves, which make up the second structure. The third structure is perpendicular to the other two. It is another system of canals, called **T-tubules,** or **transverse tubules.**

Each fiber within the cell is made up of **myofibrils (MYE oh FYE brilz)** or bundles of tiny filaments (see Figure 42). There are thick filaments made of the protein **myosin (MYE oh sin),** and thin ones made of

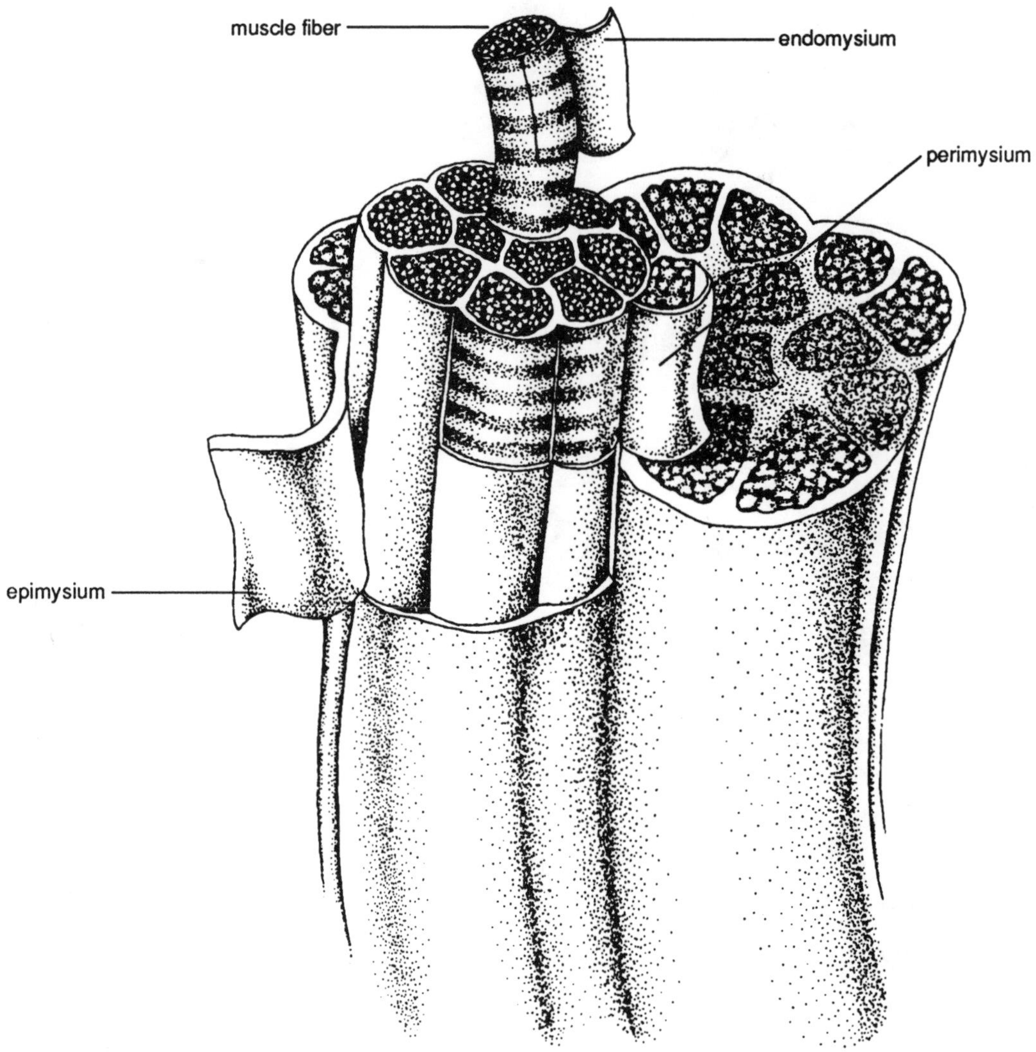

Figure 40: Muscle fiber bundle.

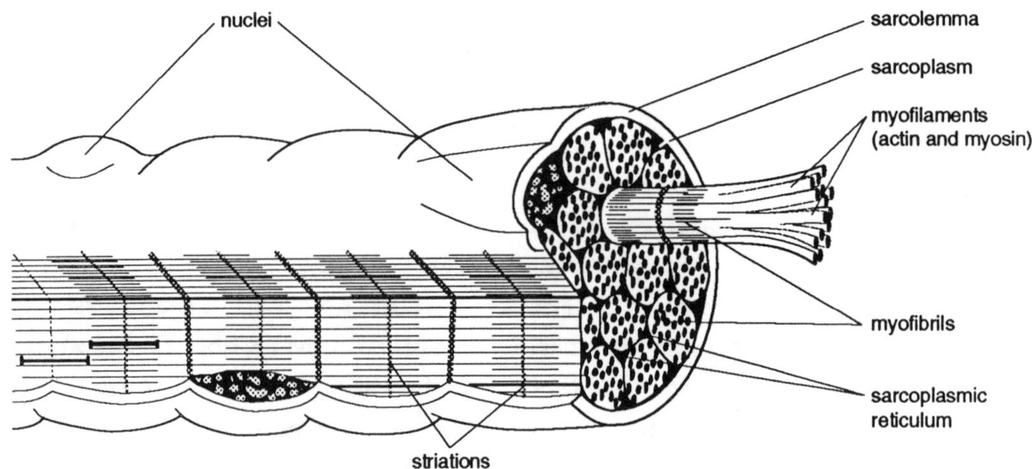

Figure 41: Part of one muscle cell.

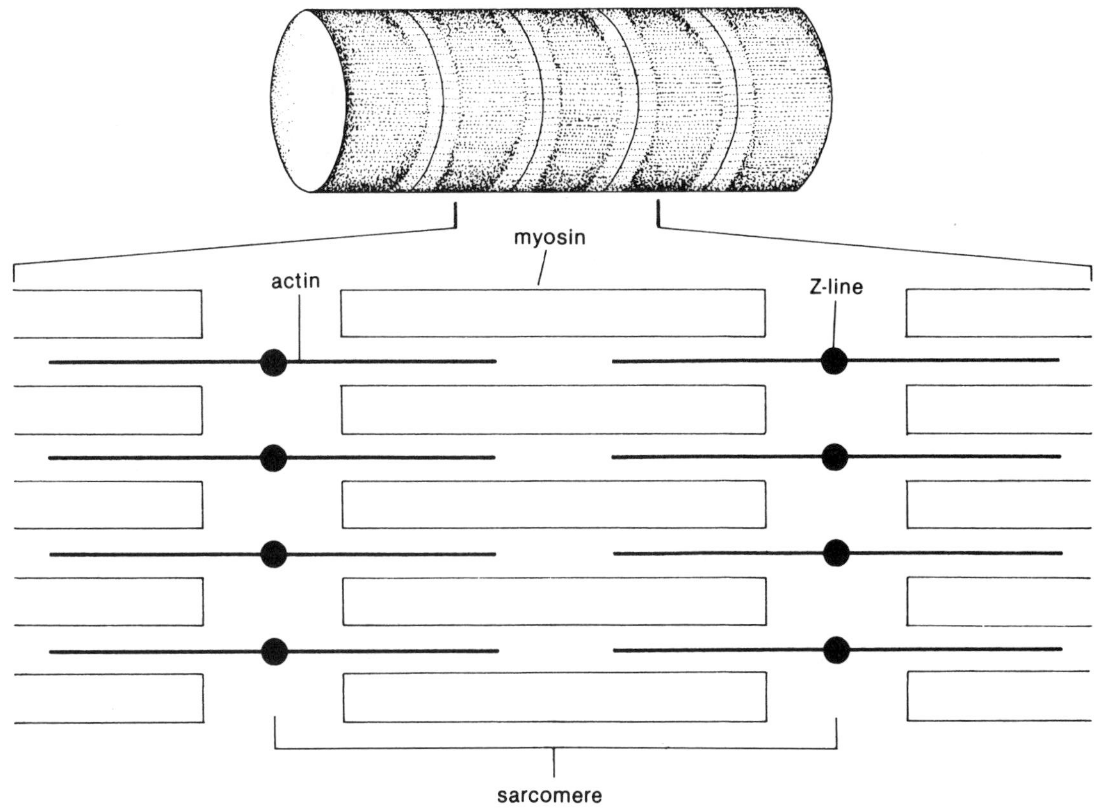

Figure 42: Diagram of myofibril structure.

another protein called **actin** (ACK tin), arranged in pairs. Each pair is joined together with extensions of the myosin filaments. These extensions are called **cross-bridges.**

Each myofibril is divided into units called **sarcomeres (SAHR koh MEERZ).** Each sarcomere has one thick and one thin filament. The sarcomeres are separated by the T-tubules, which are at right angles to them and form a boundary line called a **Z-line.** Along the Z-line are the sacs of the sarcoplasmic reticulum. These elements are all part of the mechanism of contraction, and the sarcomere is the unit of contraction. (STOP AND REVIEW, page 48.)

MUSCLE CONTRACTIONS

Muscles contract only when they are stimulated. The stimulus is an electrical impulse from a nerve or nerves associated with the muscle. This impulse moves through the muscle by changing the electrical charge of the cells from positive to negative for a fraction of a second. The cells quickly return to their original charge as the impulse moves through the muscle, but the stimulus initiates a series of activities within the muscle cells that make the muscle contract. This is what happens:

1. A motor neuron (a nerve that carries impulse *from* the brain) releases a chemical called **acetylcholine (ah SET ul KOH leen)** (ACh). ACh stimulates the muscles, and a contraction begins.
2. A microsecond later, the stimulated muscle cell releases **cholinesterase (KOH lih NES tur ays),** which destroys the acetylcholine and ends the stimulation.
3. In the meantime, the stimulus has

STOP AND REVIEW

1. Define "striated": ____
   ____
2. Name three major functions of skeletal muscles.
   a. ____
   b. ____
   c. ____
3. True/False: Tendons connect ligaments and muscles.
4. True/False: Skeletal muscles account for between 50 percent and 60 percent of body weight.
5. True/False: Each muscle cell is covered by epimysium.
6. True/False: Each muscle cell is short and fat with only a few nuclei.
7. True/False: The main body of the muscle cell is called the sarcoplasm.
8. True/False: The network of canals that contains the sacs of calcium at their ends are called T-tubes.
9. True/False: The fibers within the individual muscle cells are called myofibrils.
10. True/False: Each sarcomere contains both actin and myosin.

Fill in the blanks for questions 11 through 14.

11. Name the two types of filaments that make up the myofibrils.
    a. ____
    b. ____
12. Each filament pair is joined together by extensions called ______________________ .
13. Define the Z-line and describe the material it contains.______________________________
    ____
14. The functional unit of contraction is the ______________________________________ .

entered the muscle cell through the sarcolemma (cell membrane). Before stimulation, the cell has a high potassium content inside and a high sodium concentration outside, which gives the cell a positive charge outside and a negative charge inside. With the stimulation, sodium moves into the cell and reverses the polarization. The inside of the cell now becomes positively charged.

4. This change in polarization moves along each muscle cell. Behind this wave of polarization follows a wave of repolarization. Sodium moves out of the cell and restores the balance to its original state. Once again, the outside is positive and the inside is negative. This wave effect is called an *action potential.*

Contraction of a muscle occurs during the microsecond that it takes for the muscle cell to be stimulated and return to its original state. Contraction is also a complex activity, as follows:

1. Stimulation of the muscle cell sends a signal along the T-tubules to the sacs in the sarcoplasmic reticulum. The sacs then release calcium into the cell body. The calcium combines with a chemical called **troponin (TROH poh nin).** Troponin inhibits contraction of the cell and keeps it at rest until it is combined with calcium.
2. At the same time, **adenosine triphosphate (ah DEN ah SEEN TRY fos fayt) (ATP)** is broken down by the cell to provide energy for the contraction. This breakdown releases energy and a substance called **creatine phosphate (KREE uh teen FOS fayt)** and leaves **adenosine diphosphate (ah DEN ah SEEN DYE fos fayt) (ADP)** in place of ATP.
3. The calcium-troponin combination acts on the actin and myosin in each sarcomere of the muscle cell. The cross-bridges of myosin on the thick filaments move to attach to the thin filaments of actin at a new location, closer to the center of the sarcomere. They use the energy supplied by ATP to do this.
4. The thin filaments slide toward the center of the sarcomere, shortening the sarcomere. This occurs in each sarcomere in the muscle cell and causes a contraction.
5. The calcium returns to the sacs in the sarcoplasmic reticulum, thus reactivating the troponin and releasing the thin filaments (actin) from the cross-bridges of the thick filaments (myosin). The cross-bridges return to their original position and the sarcomeres return to their original length.
6. The muscle relaxes. Then the muscle cells use creatine phosphate to make new ATP, which will provide energy for the next contraction. (STOP AND REVIEW, page 50.)

> ***MUSCLE TONE***
>
> **Muscles are never completely relaxed, even when resting. Nerve impulses constantly flowing to the muscles maintain the fibers in a state of partial contraction, a condition known as *muscle tone.* This tone helps maintain posture, and keeps the muscles ready for action.**

Energy for Contraction. Energy released by the breakdown of ATP is the usual fuel for creating a muscle contraction. However, ATP is not always available. If a muscle is working continuously, there is no time for the cell to recreate ATP. At the same time, the supplies of resources needed to make ATP are depleted. These resources include creatine phosphate and oxygen.

To solve this problem, at least temporarily, the muscle can get energy from **glycogen (GLYE kuh JIN),** a form of carbohydrate that is stored in muscle cells. Glycogen is broken down into lactic acid and ATP to supply energy for contraction. This process uses no oxygen, yet oxygen is needed to remove the lactic acid from the muscle cell. Eventually the cell must have more oxygen. It builds up what is called an **oxygen debt.** This is one reason why strenuous activity can be continued for only a short time before the muscles tire and can no longer be persuaded to contract. Also, this mechanism

STOP AND REVIEW

1. True/False: Muscles contract only when stimulated.
2. True/False: Muscles contract due to changes in the electrical charge of their cells.
3. True/False: The nerve that stimulates a muscle to contract is called a sensory neuron.
4. True/False: During a muscle contraction, the sodium concentration increases inside the cell.
5. True/False: A muscle stimulus sends a signal along the T-tubules to the sacs at the end of the sarcoplasmic reticulum, causing them to release calcium.
6. True/False: The muscle cells use ADP as an energy source.
7. True/False: After a muscle contraction, calcium returns to the sacs in the sarcoplasmic reticulum.

explains why a person who has been exercising must take deep breaths to recover from the exertion.

During moderate exercise, when enough oxygen is available to the muscle cells, the production of ATP can keep up with the need for energy. As we have seen, ATP is broken down into ADP (adenosine diphosphate), creatine phosphate, and energy to fuel a contraction. Then the process called **oxidative phosphorylation (OCK sih DAY tiv FOS for ih LAY shun)** begins to combine ADP, creatine phosphate, and oxygen to recreate ATP. As long as there are adequate supplies of oxygen and creatine phosphate, and the contractions are not too strenuous or too close together, no oxygen debt occurs and exercise can continue.

Types and Force of Contractions. Two types of contractions are responsible for the expenditure of the major portion of muscle energy. During an **isometric (EYE suh MEH trick)** (*iso-* same, *metr-* measure or length) contraction, the length of the muscle remains the same, but the tension within the muscle increases. Isometric contraction occurs when strength is insufficient to lift a heavy weight. An **isotonic (EYE suh TAHN ick)** contraction (*tonic*-tone) contraction occurs when muscle tone remains unchanged, but the length of muscle fibers decreases. Isotonic contractions are responsible for ordinary daily movements.

The force of a particular muscle contraction, whether it is isometric or isotonic, depends on three things: how many motor neurons are acting on the muscle; how frequently those neurons stimulate the muscle cells; and how long the muscle is when stimulation begins. A single, unrepeated stimulus will cause a single, jerky contraction that is called a **twitch**. This seldom occurs in the body. If a second stimulus occurs before the muscle relaxes from an initial contraction, it is called a **summation**. In a summation, the muscle has already shortened when the second stimulus reaches it. This double contraction exerts more force on the muscle than a twitch does. If the stimuli continue to occur in rapid succession, the contraction is called a **tetanus (TET uh nus)**. This is the strongest type of contraction, because the muscle shortens with the first stimulus and then receives repeated stimuli over a short time. Most body movements are the result of several motor neurons sending a series of stimuli to several different muscles at the same time. (STOP AND REVIEW, below.)

Skeletal muscles act in groups rather than alone to move the bones. Each muscle in each group has a particular role, as a **prime mover,** a **synergist (SIN ur jist),** or an **antagonist (an TAG uh nist).**

STOP AND REVIEW

1. Name two kinds of contractions.
   a. ______________________________
   b. ______________________________
2. Name three factors which affect the strength of a muscle contraction.
   a. ______________________________
   b. ______________________________
   c. ______________________________
3. The substance that causes muscle cells to contract is ______________________ .
4. The chemical that stops muscle stimulation is______________________ .
5. Circle one: Polarization of a cell is caused by moving sodium (into/out of) the muscle cell.
6. Define action potential.______________________________
   ____
7. What chemical inhibits the contraction of a muscle cell?______________________
8. Name the two materials to which glycogen breaks down during prolonged muscle contraction.
   a. ______________________________
   b. ______________________________
9. True/False: Muscle length shortens during isotonic contraction.
10. True/False: Most body movements result from a motor neuron sending a stimulus to only one muscle.
11. Stimuli continuing in rapid succession create a contraction called a:
    a. twitch
    b. summation
    c. tetanus

As the name suggests, a prime mover exerts a major pulling force. When one or more prime movers contract, this contraction produces the actual movement of a limb.

A synergist muscle acts with the prime mover. It acts either to assist the prime mover, or to hold the moving part stable while it moves.

An antagonist moves in the opposite direction from the prime mover. Usually the antagonist relaxes as the prime mover contracts. However, it may act in another way. If the opposite muscles contract at the same time, the joint will be held rigid. An example of this dual action is found in the muscles of the knee joint when standing. Because of the weight the joint is supporting, both the antagonist and the prime mover must contract to keep the knee from bending. (STOP AND REVIEW, below.)

Specific Muscles

Muscle names are not chosen merely at random. They are associated with the location, related bones, shape, action, and/or size of the muscle. These names may be difficult to understand because they are often stated in Latin rather than English. However, if you can relate a muscle's name to these factors, it may be easier to remember where it is and what it does. For example, the external intercostal muscles are located on the outside (external part) of the body between (inter) the ribs, or costae; the quadriceps femoris is a four-part muscle (quadriceps) that originates at the thigh (femur).

There are more than 600 skeletal muscles in the human body, but only the major muscles will be covered here. A muscle that induces a precise movement, such as raising an eyebrow or opening an eye, is much smaller and has fewer muscle fibers than a muscle that moves a large limb. This is why there are more major muscles in the face than in the limbs.

Facial Muscles. Table 11 lists just a few of the muscles that govern facial expressions, eyesight, speech, and all the other small movements that the human face makes constantly.

You use the **epicranius (EP ih KRAY nee us)** to express surprise and puzzlement. It stretches from the frontal bone of the cranium back to the occipital bone. The front part of this muscle, called the **frontalis (frun**

STOP AND REVIEW

1. Skeletal muscles work in concert to move bones. Name three possible roles a muscle may play in movement.

   a. ______________________________

   b. ______________________________

   c. ______________________________

2. Name a muscle that either helps the prime mover or holds the moving part stable during movement. ______________________________

3. Which muscles contract when a joint is held stable? ______________________________

4. Circle one: Muscles produce movement by (pushing/pulling) on bones.

TAH lis), raises the eyebrows and wrinkles the forehead. The rear, or **occipitalis (ock SIP ih TAH lis),** relaxes those features again (see Figure 43).

The **orbicularis oculi (or BICK yoo LAH ris OCK yoo lye)** muscles (see Figure 43) surround the eye sockets and pass beneath the eyelids. These muscles control both involuntary and deliberate closing of the eyes.

The **levator palpebrae superioris (leh VAY tur pal PEE bree soo peer ee OH ris)** muscles have the opposite effect. They open the eyes both when you wake up and whenever you blink. Each one is a long, thin muscle attached to the sphenoid bone at one end and the eyelid at the other.

The **orbicularis oris (OH ris)** surrounds the mouth and joins other muscles of the mouth including the **buccinator (BUCK sih NAY tur).** This muscle causes you to purse your lips for a kiss or a pout. The **zygomatic muscle** is attached to the zygomatic bone in the cheek. This muscle raises the corner of your mouth for a smile or a laugh.

The buccinator forms the side wall of the mouth. It keeps the cheek in its proper place against the teeth, and keeps food in the teeth as you chew.

The **platysma (plah TIZ muh),** at the front of the neck, stretches from the front of the chest to the lower jaw. It pulls down the lower jaw, the lower lip, and the corners of the mouth, and also wrinkles the skin of the neck.

The **rectus** muscles, superior, inferior, lateral, and medial, move the eye sideways and up and down. They are attached to the eyeball itself (see Figure 44). The superior and inferior oblique muscles are also in the eye socket, but are attached to the bone above and below the eye (superior above and inferior below). Their function is to rotate or roll the eyes. All six of these muscles are attached to the sphenoid bone at the other end. They work together to position the eyes so that you can look in any direction.

The **masseter (mah SEE tur)** (see Figure 43) lifts the lower jaw (mandible bone). It is located in front of the ear and above the jaw. The temporal muscle works with the masse-

Table 11: Facial Muscles

Muscle / Location	Number
Epicranus	
top of head	1 (2 parts)
Orbicularis oculi	
around eye	2
Levator palpebrae superioris	
beneath eyelid	2
Orbicularis oris	
around mouth	1
Zygomatic	
inside of cheek	2
Buccinator	
lower cheek	2
Platysma	
front of neck	2
Superior, inferior, lateral and medial rectus	
top, bottom, side and center of eye socket	8 (2 of each)
Superior and inferior obliques	
center of eye socket, top and bottom	4 (2 of each)
Masseter	
in front of ear	2
Temporal	
over temporal bone	2
Pterygoid	
at junction of jaw bones	4

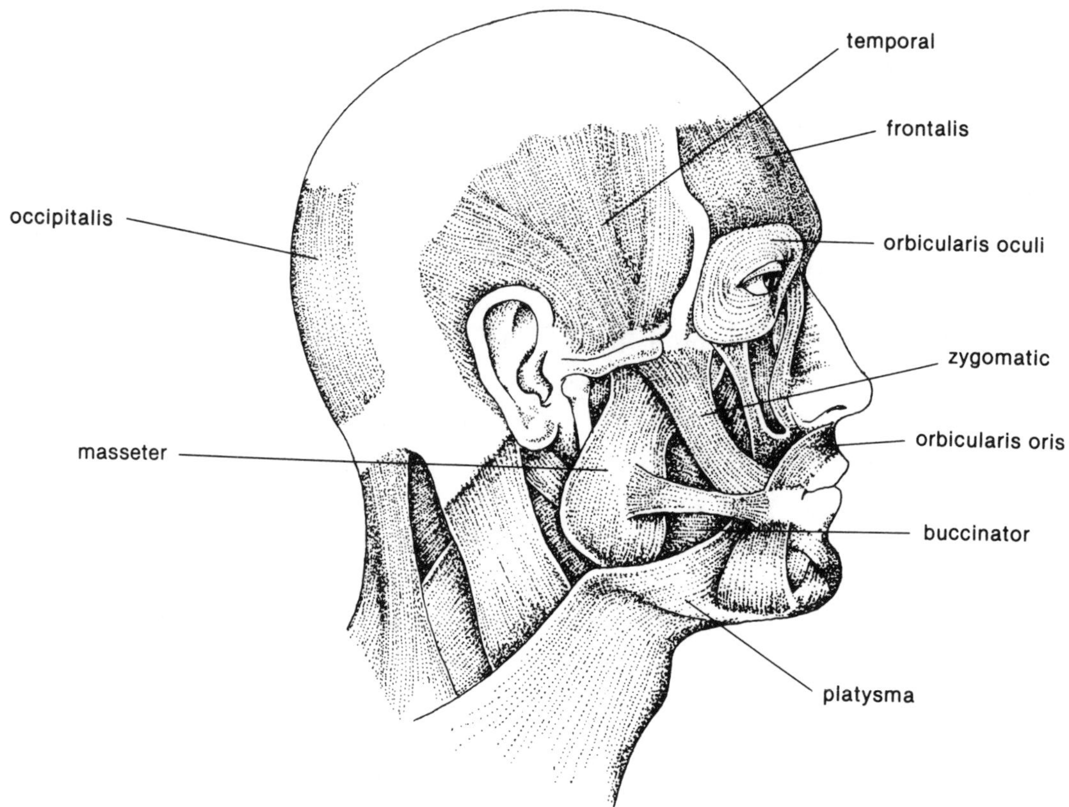

Figure 43: Facial muscles.

ter (see Figure 45). Its position is above the temporal bone and farther back on the cranium. The four **pterygoid (TERR ih goyd) muscles** also move the lower jaw, but they move it from side to side. The upper jaw remains stable as these eight muscles function in chewing and opening the mouth to enable speech. (STOP AND REVIEW, page 56.)

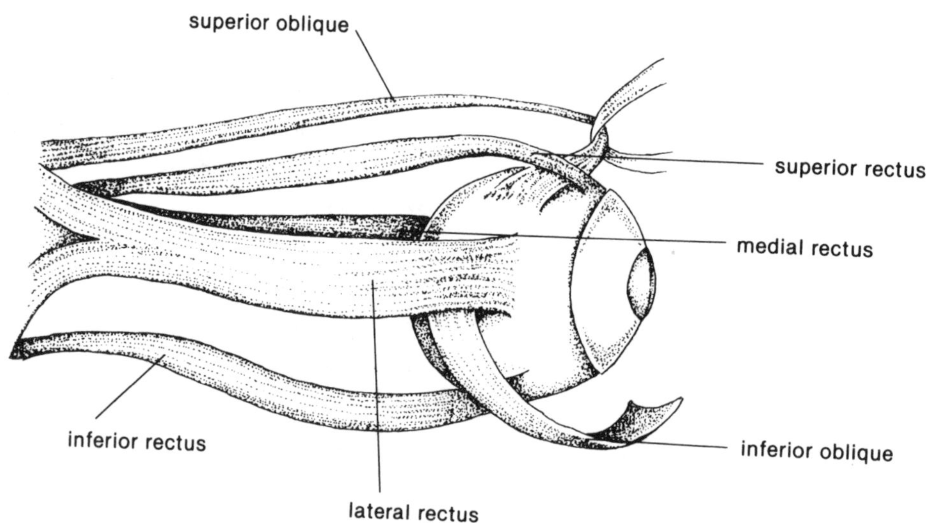

Figure 44: Rectus muscles of the eye.

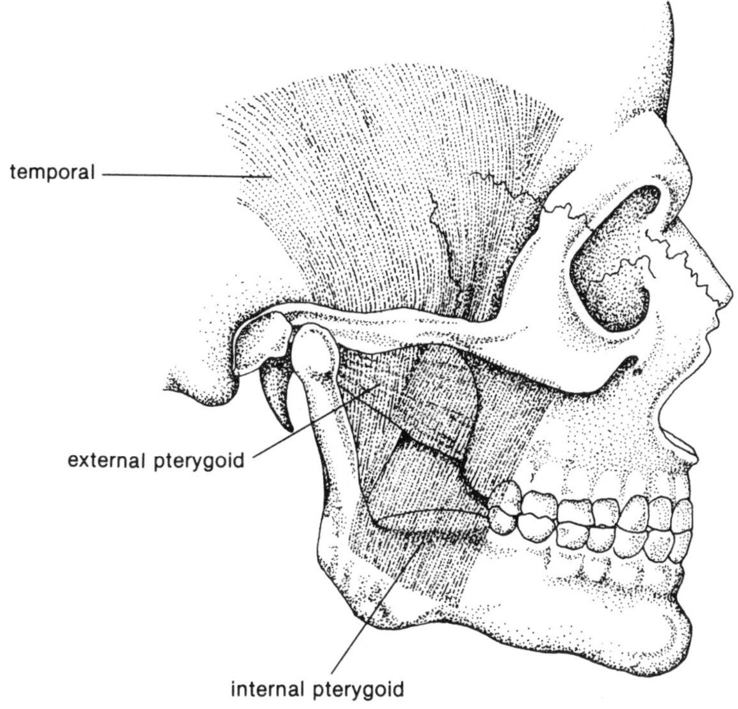

Figure 45: Muscles that move the mandible.

Table 12: Head and Neck Muscles

Semispinalis capitis	
back of neck	2
Sternocleidomastoid	
front of neck	2

Head and Neck Muscles. These muscles, though located in the neck, move the head (see Table 12). The two **semispinalis capitis (SEM ee spye NAH lis KAP ih tis)** muscles (see Figure 46) are in the back of the neck, between the occipital bone and the sixth thoracic vertebra vertebra. When they contract, they move the head backward and to the sides. The **sternocleidomastoids (STUR noh klye doh MAS toyds)** (see Figure 47) pull the head forward and to the sides. They are located in the front of the neck, and stretch from the sternum and clavicle to the mastoid bone.

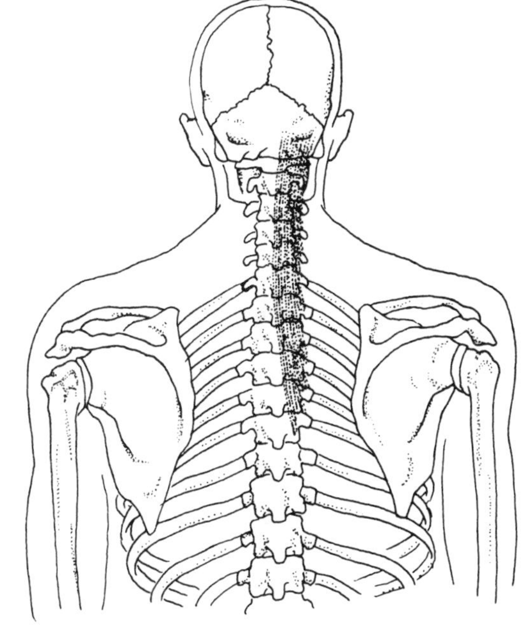

Figure 46. Semispinalis capitis.

Shoulder and Arm Muscles. The **trapezius (trah PEE zee us)** (see Figure 48) is a large

STOP AND REVIEW

1. Circle the number of muscles in the human body.
   a. 206
   b. 340
   c. more than 600
2. Circle the action that requires more muscles than the others.
   a. smiling
   b. standing
   c. raising an eyebrow
   d. nodding the head
3. Circle the "kissing" muscle.
   a. epicranius
   b. orbicularis oris
   c. masseter
   d. zygomatic
   e. orbicularis oculi
4. Circle the muscles you use in eating.
   a. superior rectus
   b. pterygoid
   c. zygomatic
   d. platysma
   e. masseter
   f. buccinator
   g. temporal

triangular muscle that covers the shoulder blade (scapula) and stretches up into the neck and down to the last (twelfth) thoracic vertebra. This muscle works with the other shoulder muscles in many movements; it also acts alone to draw the scapula toward the spine and up, for example, in shrugging the shoulders.

The **pectoralis (PECK toh RAH lis) major** (see Figure 49) covers the front of the chest from the sternum (breastbone), and clavicle (collar bone), and also attaches to the humerus (upper arm bone). It is shaped like a fan. It works to adduct the arm, that is, to lower the arm after it has been raised. This muscle also rotates the arm inward and draws it across the chest.

The **latissimus dorsi (lah TIS ih mus**

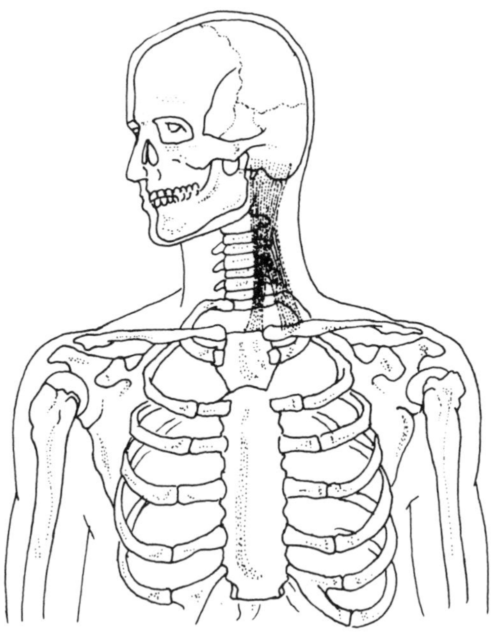

Figure 47: Sternocleidomastoid.

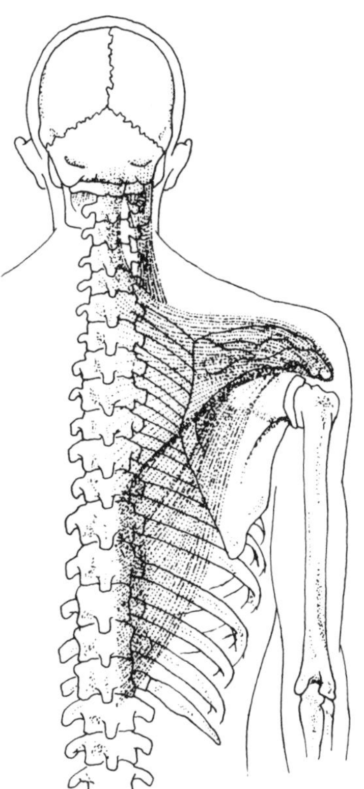

Figure 48: Trapezius.

DOR sye) (see Figure 50) covers the lower back from the hip and is attached to the spine up to the seventh thoracic vertebra. Its top is under the trapezius. On the other side, it is twisted and attaches to the underside of the humerus. This large muscle works with the pectoralis major to move the upper arm. It is also considered an abdominal muscle (see Table 17).

Table 13: Shoulder and Arm Muscles

Trapezius	
over shoulder blade	2
Pectoralis major	
front of chest	2
Latissimus dorsi	
lower back	2
Deltoid	
top of arm	2
Biceps brachii and biceps brachialis	
front of upper arm	4
Triceps brachii	
back of upper arm	2

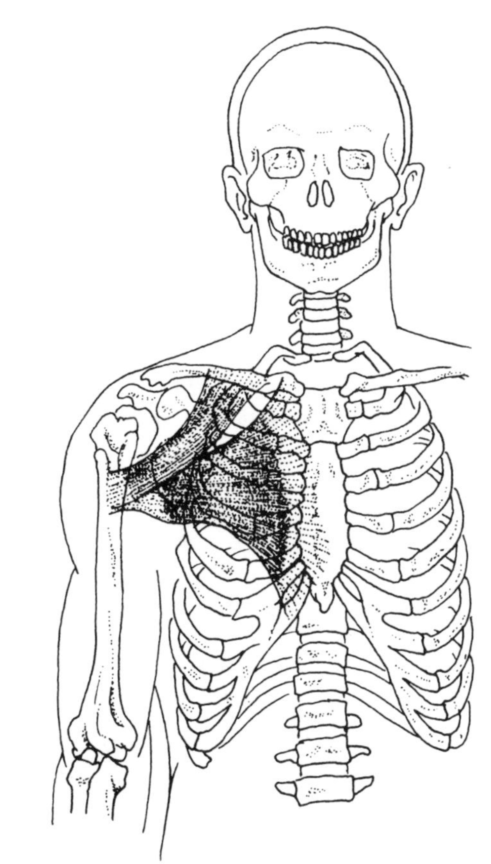

Figure 49: Pectoralis major.

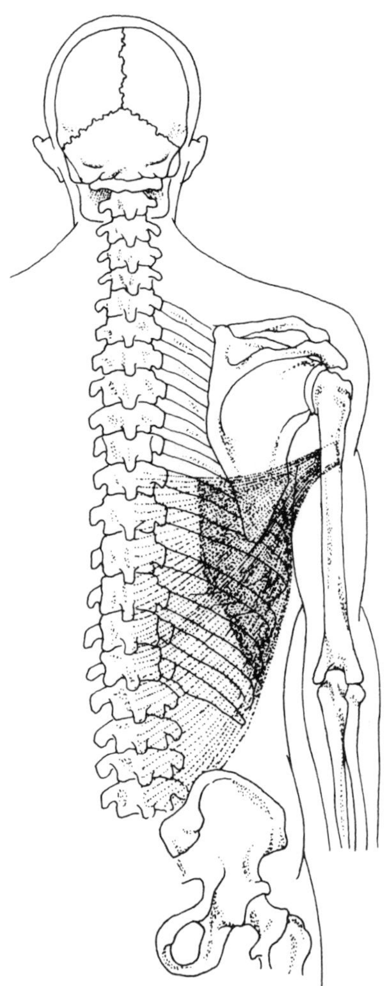

Figure 50: Latissimus dorsi.

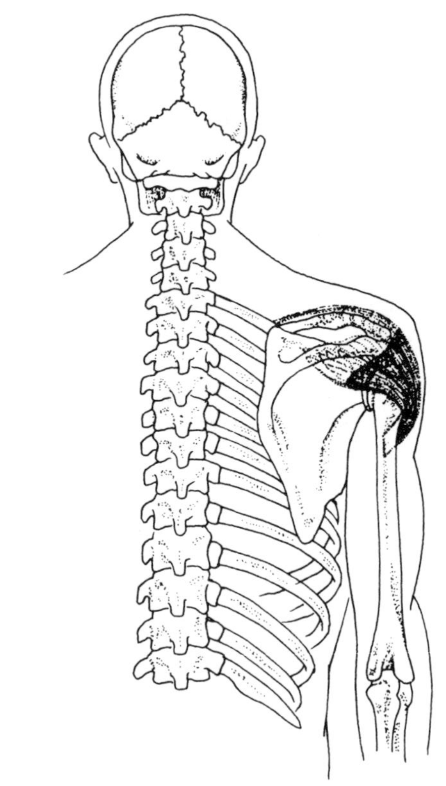

Figure 51: Deltoid.

The **deltoid (DEL toyd)** (see Figure 51) muscle is attached to the clavicle in the front of the shoulder, the scapula in the back, and to the humerus. It covers the top of the shoulder, and abducts the arm, or moves it up so that it is level with the shoulder and straight out.

Two muscles, the **biceps brachii (BRAY kee eye)** and the **brachialis (BRAY kee AY lis)** (see Figures 52 and 53), act together to **flex** (bend) the lower arm at the elbow. The biceps brachii attaches to the scapula (shoulder) and the radius (lower arm), while the brachialis attaches to the humerus (upper arm) and the ulna (lower arm).

The **triceps brachii** (see Figure 54) is attached to the shoulder, upper arm, and

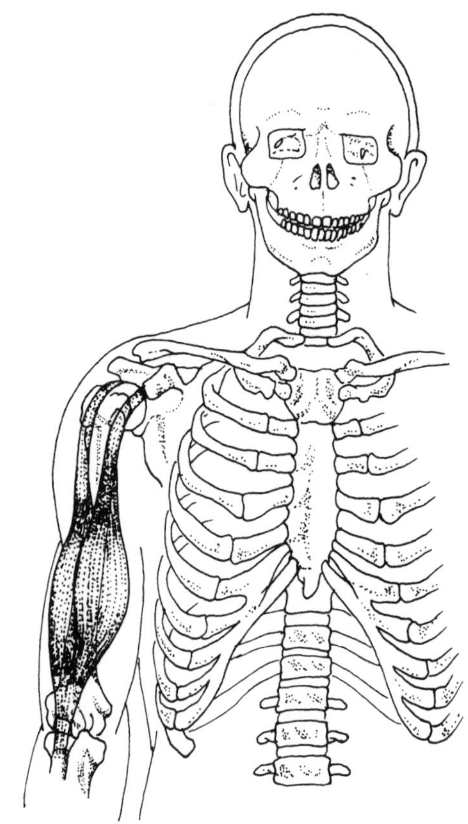

Figure 52: Biceps brachii.

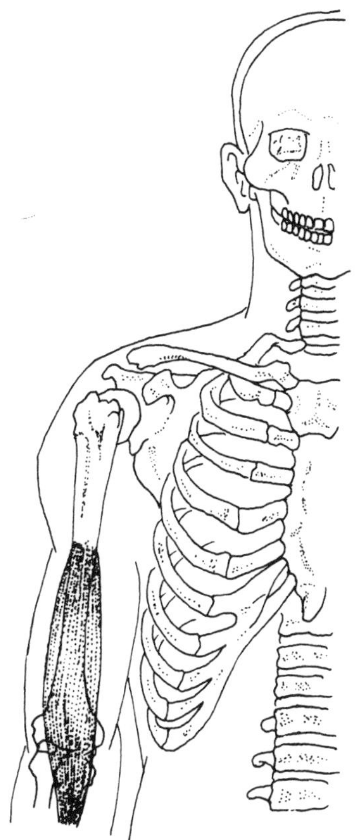

Figure 53: Brachialis.

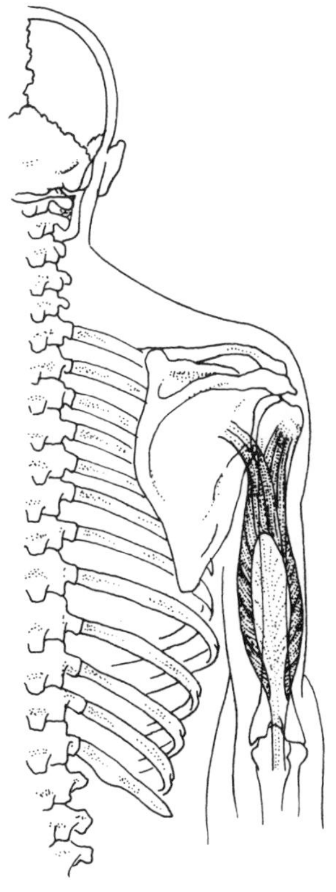

Figure 54: Triceps brachii.

Table 14: Review of Five Major Movements

Flexion	move forward or bend from a resting position
Extension	return from flexion to a resting position
Abduction	move sideways from center
Adduction	return from abduction to center
Rotation	pivot

lower arm. It extends the arm, which is the opposite function from that of the biceps brachii and the brachialis. Table 14 reviews the major movements of muscles.

Wrist and Hand Muscles. The muscles that flex and extend the hand, wrist and fingers stretch from the area around the elbow all the way to the hand (see Figure 55 and Table 15). There are many other smaller muscles in the hand that control the precise movements of hands and fingers in finely detailed work.

The **flexor carpi radialis (FLECK sur kahr pye ray dee AY lis)** is attached to the humerus at the elbow and to the base of the second metacarpal at the other end. It flexes both the forearm and the hand. The **palmaris longus (pal MAY ris LONG gus)** is also attached to the humerus, but spreads to cover the entire hand and is attached to the four metacarpals of the palm. It flexes the hand only.

The **flexor carpi ulnaris (ul NAY ris)** is attached to both the humerus and the ulna at the elbow, and to the wrist and the metacarpals at the hand. It both flexes and adducts the hand.

The **extensor carpi radialis longus (eck STEN sur)** attaches to the humerus and the second metacarpal, and is located along the length of the radius. Its functions are to return the flexed hand to rest position (extension) and to abduct the hand toward

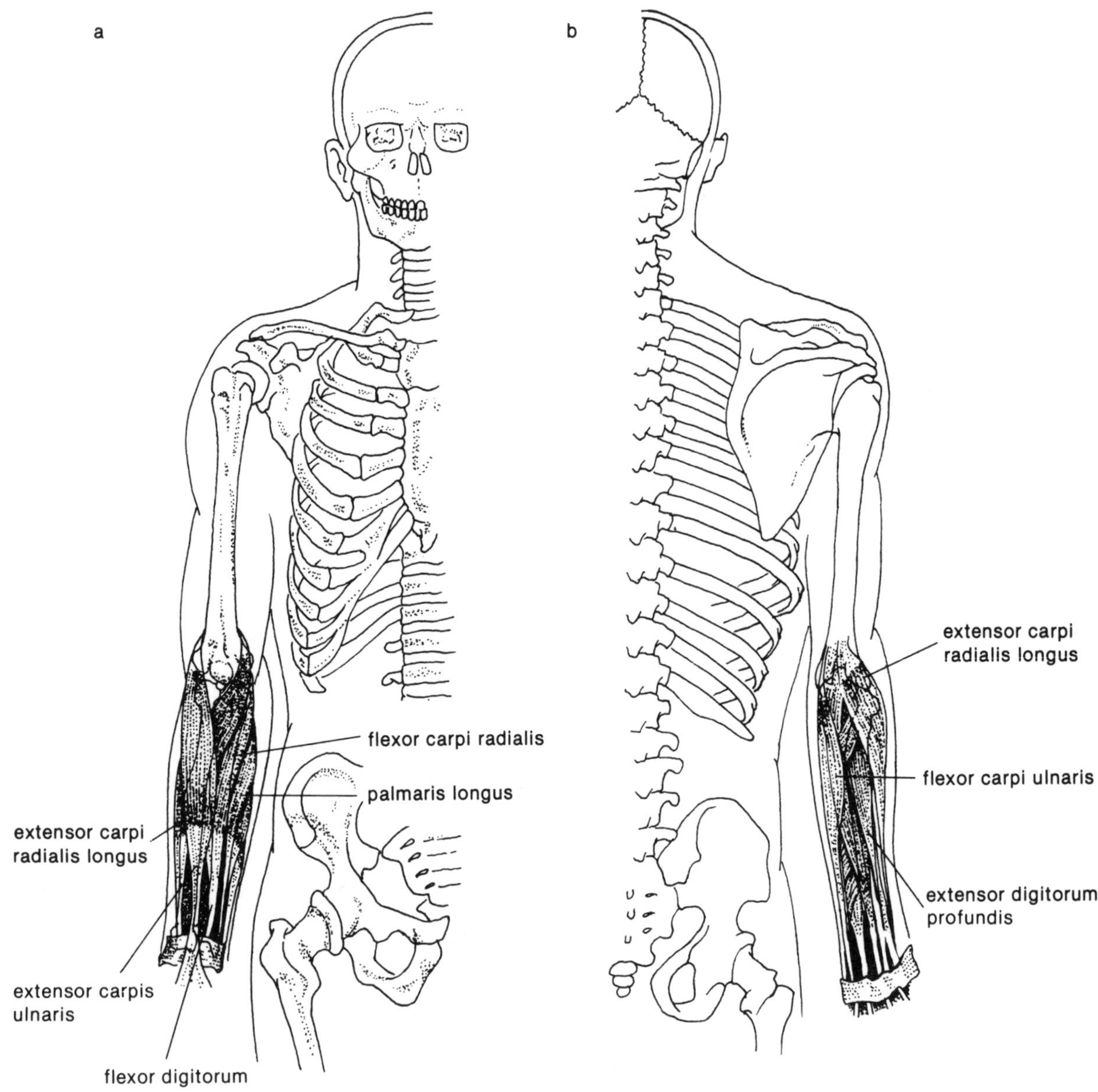

Figure 55: Anterior (a) and posterior (b) views of the forearm muscles.

the thumb.

The **extensor carpi ulnaris** is attached to the humerus and the ulna at the elbow, and to the base of the fifth metacarpal (little finger side). This muscle extends the hand and moves it toward the little finger side. This second function, called *adduction,* is the opposite of abduction, the function of the extensor carpi radialis longus.

As their names indicate, the next three muscles move the fingers (or digits). The **flexor digitorum profundus (dij ih TOH rum pro FUN dis)** is located close to the bone on the inside of the arm. The **flexor digitorum,** sometimes called the **flexor digitorum superficialis (SOO pur fish ee AY lis)** is above it. The **extensor digitorum** is on the outside of the arm. (STOP AND REVIEW, page 62)

Respiration Muscles. The respiratory muscles work together to expand and contract the

Table 15: Wrist and Hand Muscles

Muscle	
Flexor carpi radialis	
upper arm to hand	2
Palmaris longus	
upper arm to entire palm	2
Flexor carpi ulnaris	
upper arm to lower arm to wrist	2
Extensor carpi radialis longus	
upper arm to hand	2
Extensor carpi ulnaris	
upper and lower arm to hand	2
Flexor digitorum	
upper and lower arm to middle of fingers	2
Flexor digitorum profundus	
lower arm to fingertips	2
Extensor digitorum	
upper and lower arm to middle fingers	2
Flexor digitorum profoundus	
lower arm to fingertips	2
Extensor digitorum	
upper arm to middle of fingers	2

Table 16: Respiration Muscles

Muscle	
Diaphragm	
lower chest, below lungs and above abdominal cavity	1
External intercostals	
between ribs on outside	22
Internal intercostals	
between ribs on inside	22

the chest during inhalation and exhalation (see Table 16).

The **diaphragm (DYE uh FRAM)** is a large, dome-shaped muscle that separates the thorax, or chest, from the abdomen. It is located just below the lungs (see Figure 56). This muscle allows the chest to expand when you inhale. The intercostal muscles, internal and external, work with the diaphragm as you breathe (see Figure 57). The **external intercostals (IN tur KOS tulz)** enlarge the chest by moving the ribs up. The **internal intercostals** contract the chest as

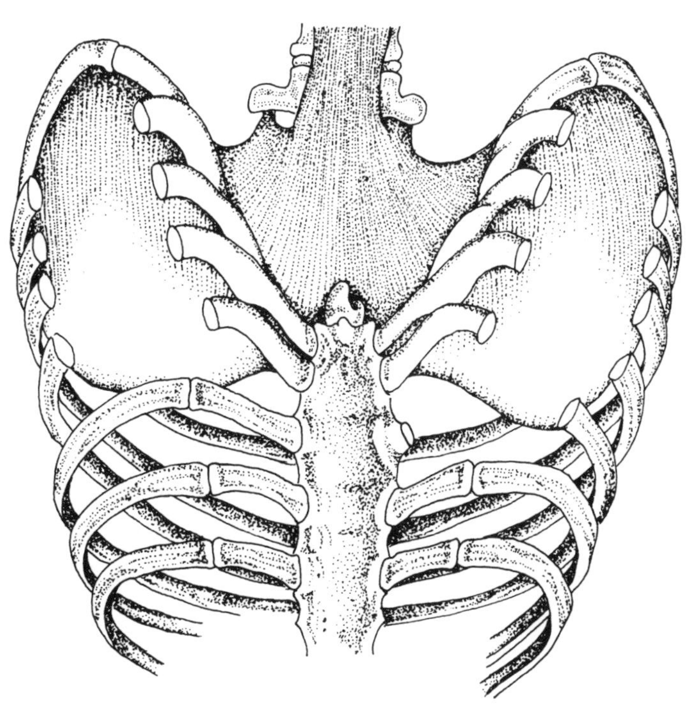

Figure 56. Diaphragm.

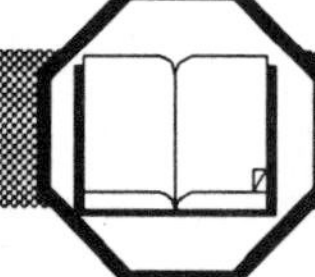

STOP AND REVIEW

Fill in the blanks for questions 1 through 5.

1. Place the letter *A* next to the muscles found in the front of the neck. Place the letter *P* next to those found in the back of the next.

   a. semispinalis capitis ______________________

   b. sternocleidomastoid______________________

   c. buccinator ______________________

   d. pterygoid ______________________

2. The muscles that move the head are located in the ______________________ .

3. The muscle of question 1 that is attached to the clavicle is the______________________ .

4. The three large muscles that cover (a) the shoulder blade, (b) the front of the chest, and (c) the lower back are called, respectively:

   a. ______________________

   b. ______________________

   c. ______________________

5. The arm muscle that is also considered an abdominal muscle is called the____________
   ______________________ .

6. Circle the names of the two muscles that act together to flex the lower arm at the elbow.

   a. deltoid

   b. brachialis

   c. pectoralis major

   d. biceps brachii

7. Define each of these major movements:

   a. flexion ______________________
   ____

   b. extension ______________________
   ____

   c. abduction ______________________
   ____

   d. adduction ______________________
   ____

   e. rotation______________________
   ____

(continued next page)

STOP AND REVIEW

8. Name the part of the body moved by these muscles:
   a. flexor digitorum profundus ______________________
   b. flexor digitorum______________________
   c. extensor digitorum ______________________
9. Identify the structures labeled on the diagrams below.
   a. ______________________
   b. ______________________
   c. ______________________
   d. ______________________
   e. ______________________

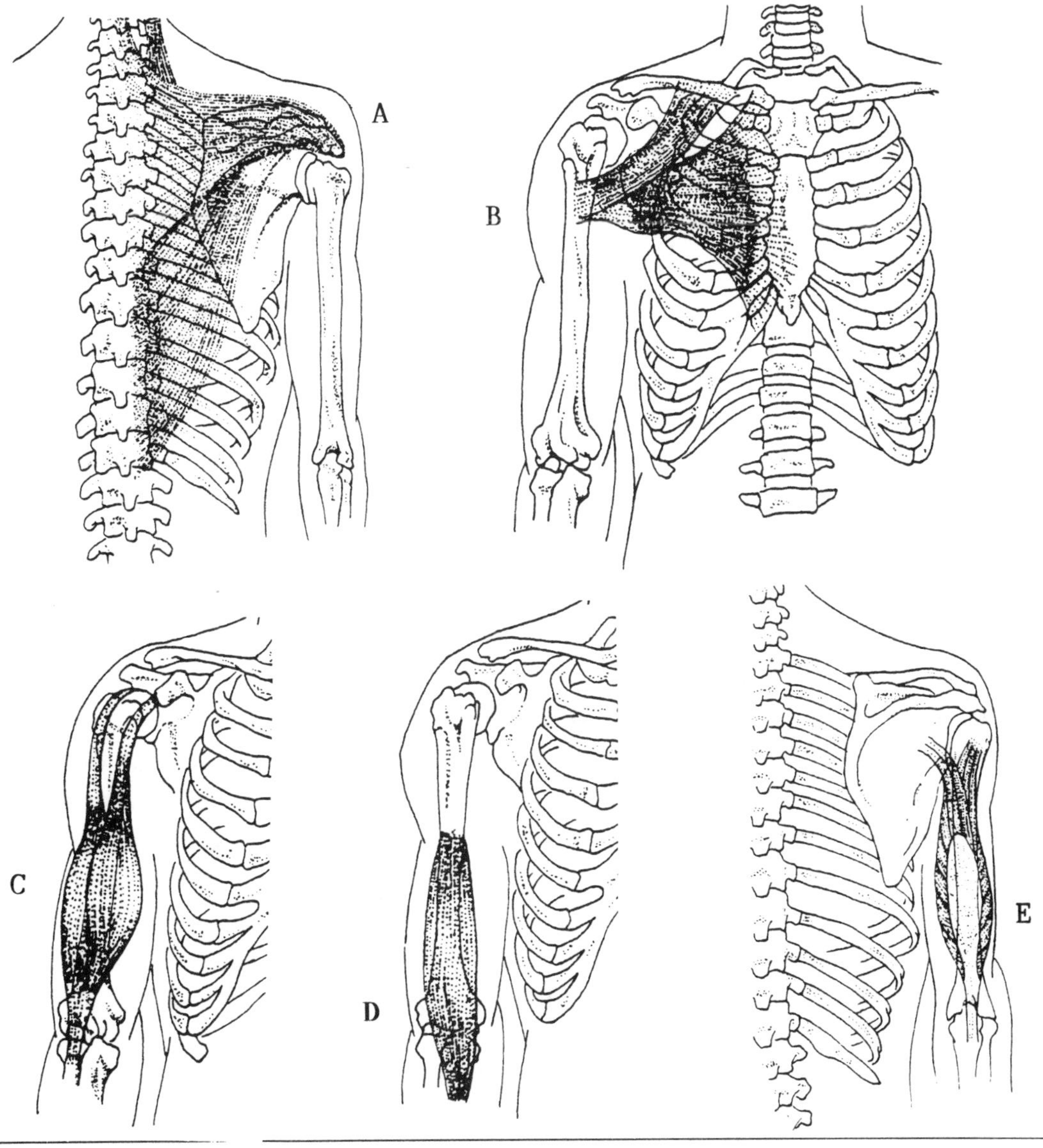

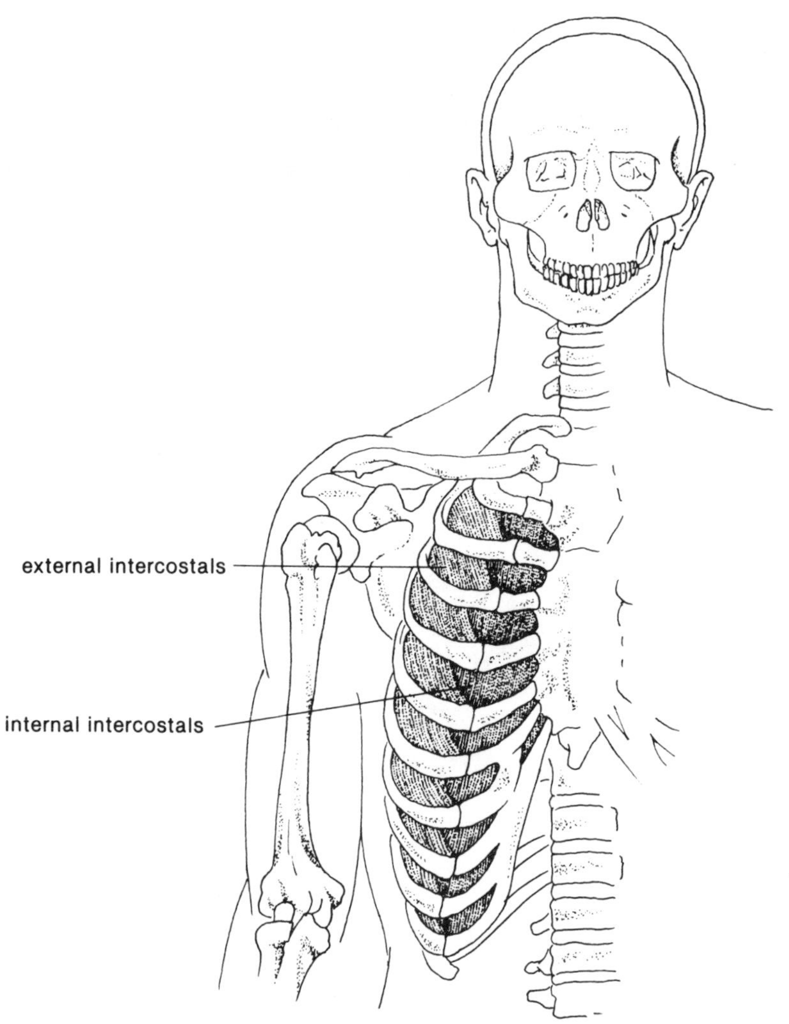

Figure 57: Intercostal muscles.

you exhale, by moving the ribs back to their original position.

Abdominal Muscles. The abdominal muscles work together to hold the organs of the abdominal cavity inside and to compress the cavity (see Table 17 and Figure 58). They have three other important functions. One is to help in moving waste out of the body through urination and defecation (moving the bowels). The second (in women only) is to help move a fetus through the birth canal during delivery. The third is to move the spinal column so that you can bend over.

The **latissimus dorsi** is the muscle located in the back of the abdominal cavity, inside the spine. The sides of the cavity are made up of three layers of muscles. These are the **external obliques (oh BLEEKS)** on the outside, the **internal obliques** in the middle, and the **transverse abdominis (ab DOM ih nis)** on the inside. (Be careful not to confuse these abdominal obliques with the superior and inferior obliques of the eye.) The **rectus abdominis** is formed by an extension of those three layers, and it is located at the front of the abdominal cavity. (STOP AND REVIEW, page 65.)

STOP AND REVIEW

1. Circle the name of the largest of the following muscles.
   a. latissimus dorsi
   b. external intercostal
   c. transverse abdominis
   d. diaphragm
2. Circle the name of the muscle(s) that contract the chest as you exhale.
   a. diaphragm
   b. external oblique
   c. transverse abdominis
   d. external intercostal
   e. internal intercostal
3. Name the functions of the abdominal muscles.
   a. ______________________________
   b. ______________________________
   c. ______________________________
   d. ______________________________(women only)
4. The rectus abdominis is formed by an extension of:
   a. ______________________________
   b. ______________________________
   c. ______________________________
5. What movement is controlled by contraction of the abdominal muscles? ______________
   ____

Hip and Leg Muscles. These muscles work together to produce movement of the buttocks and lower extremities (see Table 18). The **gluteus maximus (GLOO tee us MACK sih mus)** (see Figure 59) is the muscle you sit on. Its function is to extend the thigh and **rotate** the thigh outward. It is important in running and climbing.

The **adductor longus (ad DUCK tur)** is attached to the pubic bone and stretches to the lower leg in the front. It adducts the thigh.

The **quadriceps femoris (KWAH drih seps FEM oh ris)** (see Figure 60) has four parts. It stretches from the front of the hip to the tibia in front of the lower leg, and serves

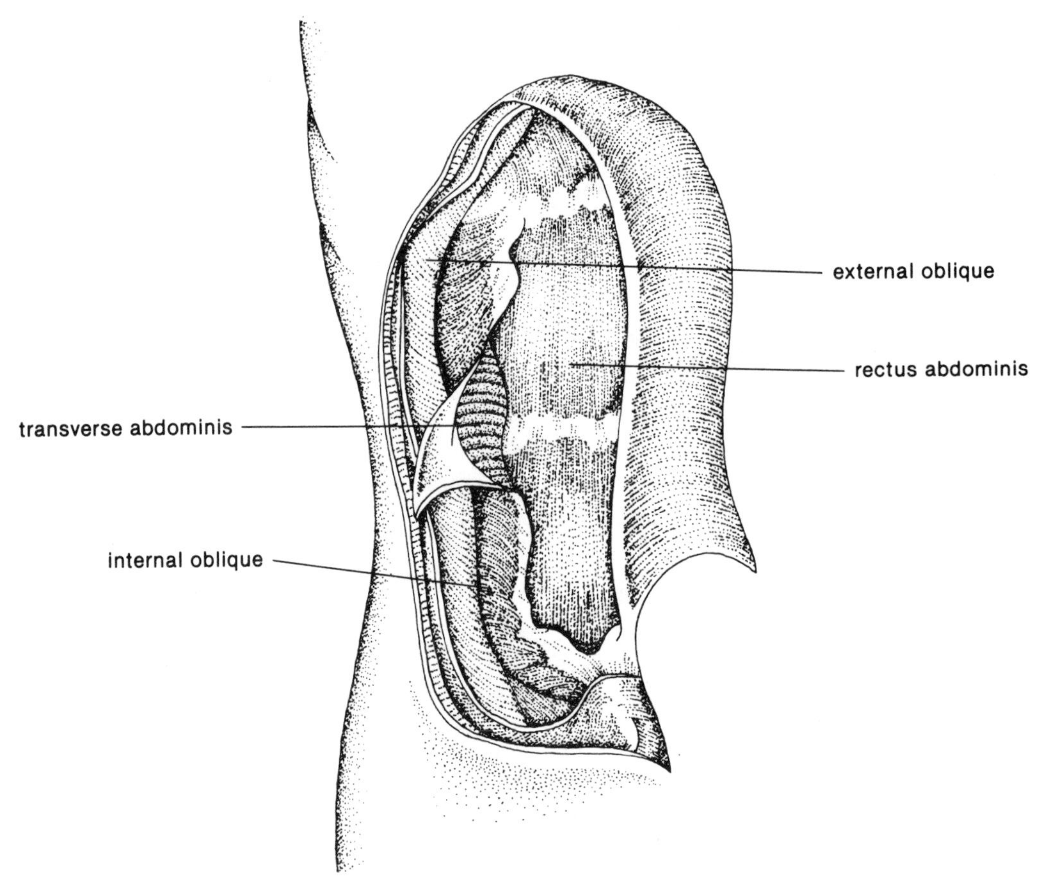

Figure 58. Muscles of abdominal wall.

Table 17: Abdominal Muscles

Muscle	
External oblique	
outer layer, sides of abdomen	2
Internal oblique	
middle layer, sides of abdomen	2
Transverse abdominis	
inner layer, sides of abdomen	2
Rectus abdominis	
front of abdomen	2
Latissimus dorsi	
back of abdominal cavity	2

Table 18: Hip and Leg Muscles

Muscle	
Gluteus maximus	
buttock	2
Adductor longus	
surface of lower leg	2
Quadriceps femoris	
front of thigh	2 (4 parts)
Sartorius	
front of thigh	2
Hamstrings	
back of thigh	2 (3 parts)
Gastrocnemius	
back of lower leg	2
Soleus	
back of lower leg	2
Tibialis anterior	
front of lower leg	2

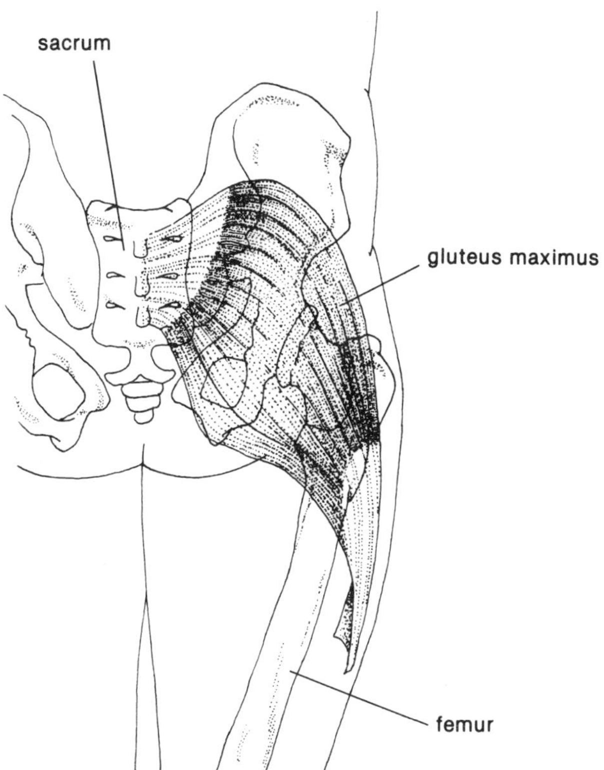

Figure 59: Gluteus maximus.

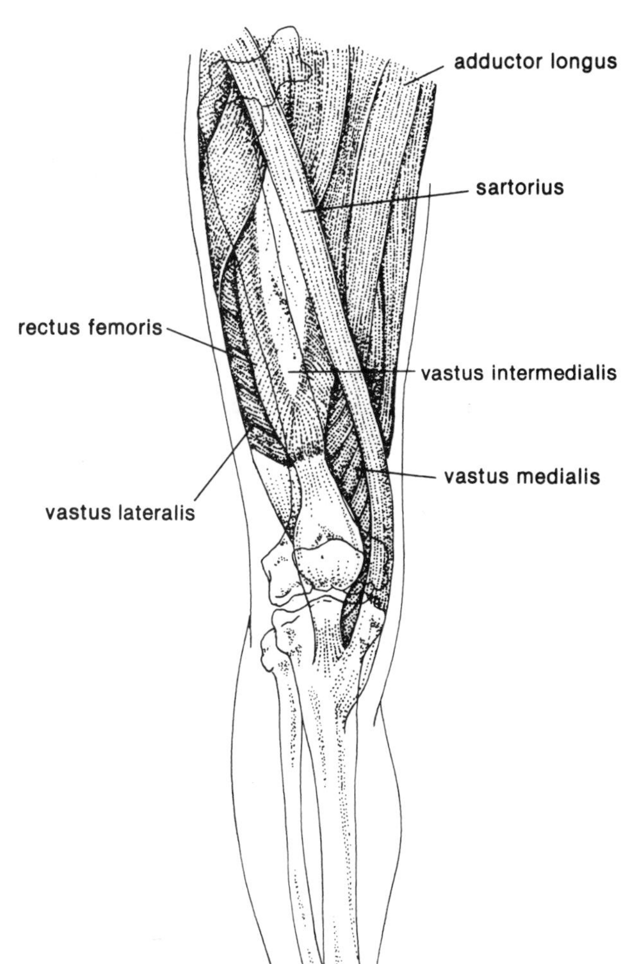

Figure 60: Anterior view of upper leg muscles (quadriceps femoris).

to extend the lower leg and flex the thigh. The parts are named rectus femoris, **vastus lateralis (VAS tus LAT ur AY is), vastus medialis,** and **vastus intermedius (IN tur MEE dee us).**

The hamstrings (see Figure 61) are found at the back of the thigh. They originate in the ischium, extend down the back of the thigh, and are anchored to the tibia and fibula in the rear of the lower leg. These muscles flex the lower leg and extend the thigh. The three parts of the hamstring are named the biceps femoris, **semitendinosus (SEM ee ten di NO sus)** and **semimembranosus (SEM ee mem bray NO sus).**

The **sartorius (sar TOR ee us)** attaches to the front of the hip, goes across the front of the thigh at an angle, and attaches to the tibia below the knee joint. This muscle flexes and adducts the lower leg. Its position across the thigh makes it possible to cross the legs.

The **gastrocnemius (GAS trok NEE mee us)** and the **soleus (SOH lee us)** together form the calf of the leg (see Figure 62). The gastrocnemius is attached to the thigh bone and the ankle, while the soleus begins on the lower leg beneath the gastrocnemius and ends on the opposite side of the ankle. These two muscles extend the foot.

STOP AND REVIEW

1. Name the two muscles in the leg that have more than one part.

   a. ______________________________

   b. ______________________________

2. Name two functions of the gluteus maximus muscle.

   a. ______________________________

   b. ______________________________

3. Identify the muscles labeled on the diagram below.

   a. ______________________________

   b. ______________________________

   c. ______________________________

   d. ______________________________

   e. ______________________________

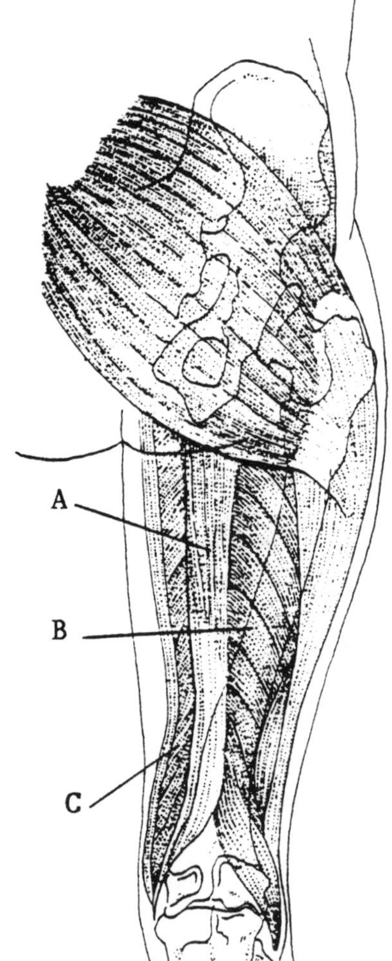

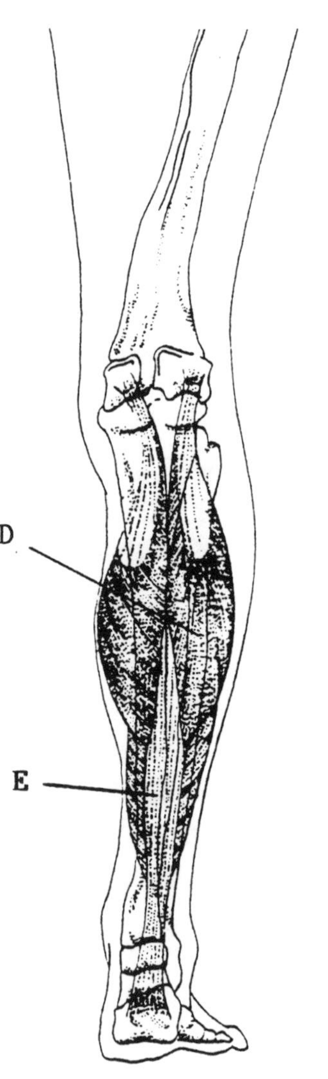

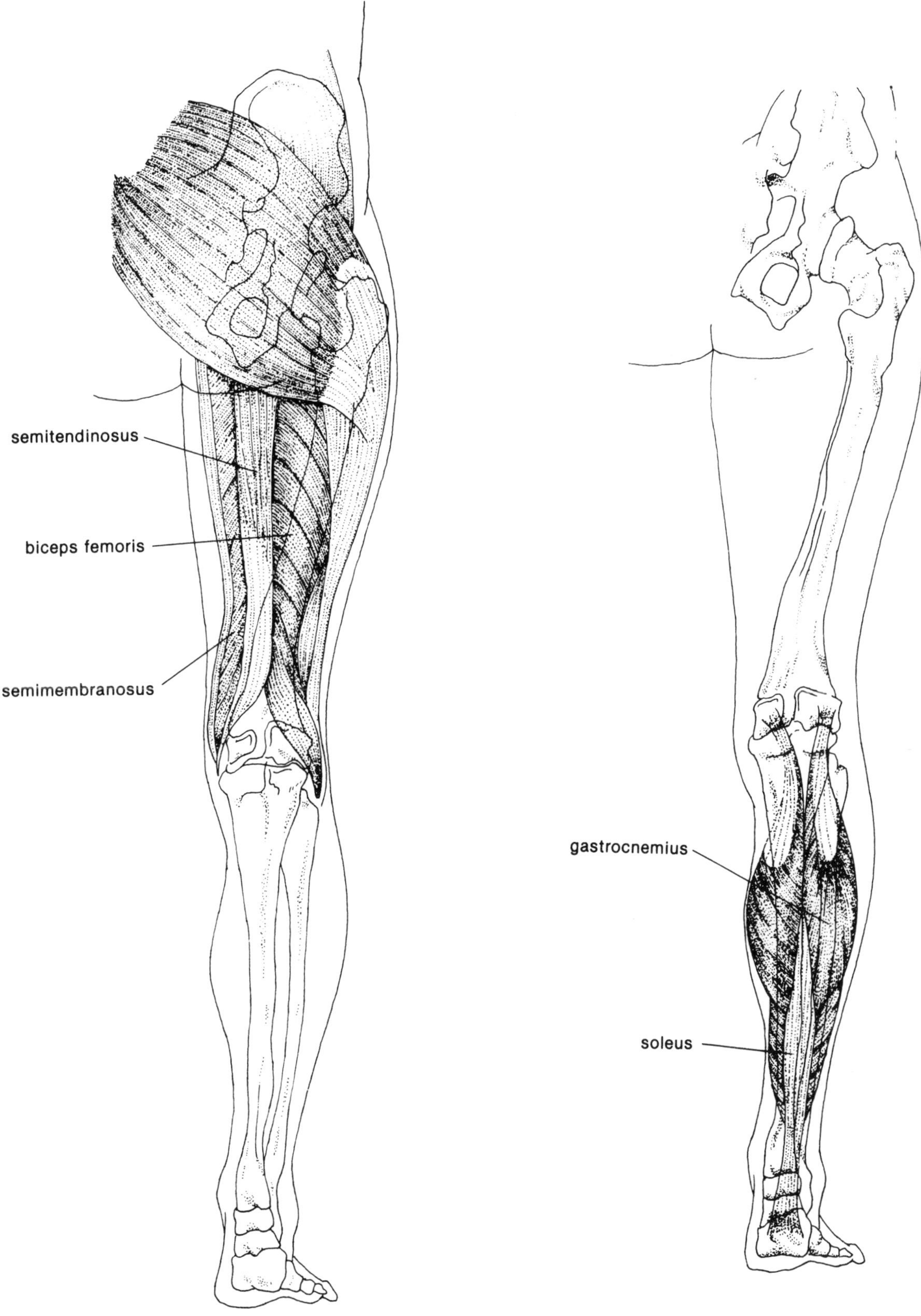

Figure 61: Posterior view of upper leg muscles (hamstrings).

Figure 62: Posterior view of lower leg muscles.

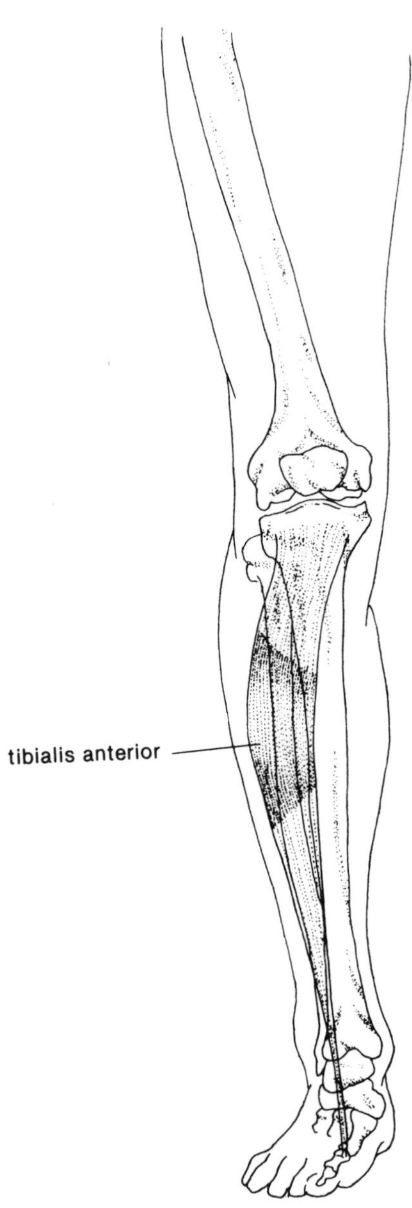

Figure 63: Tibialis anterior.

The **tibialis anterior (TIB ee AY lis an TEER ee ur)** (see Figure 63) begins at the tibia on the front of the lower leg and goes to the metatarsal of the big toe. Its function is to flex the foot.

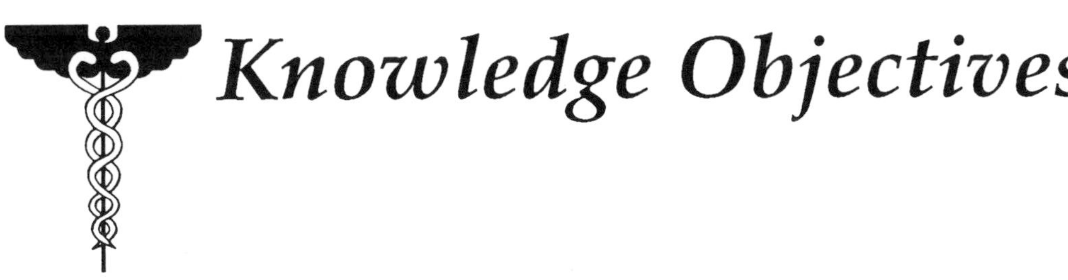

Knowledge Objectives

After completing this chapter, you should be able to:

Injuries

- describe characteristics of the different types of fractures
- describe two methods used to return bones to their normal position and alignment
- define and describe the terms *sprain, strain,* and *dislocation*

Joint Diseases

- describe several common joint disorders

Bone Diseases

- describe diseases that directly affect the bones

Muscle Diseases

- describe the pathologies of several muscle diseases

Connective Tissue Diseases

- define and describe a collagen disease

CHAPTER 3

Injuries, Diseases, and Disorders of the Musculoskeletal System

INTRODUCTION

So far, we have seen the parts that make up the musculoskeletal system. It is obvious that these parts—the bones, the joints, the muscles, and the connective tissues that hold them together—depend on each other and on the rest of the body's systems to function. If any one of the parts becomes injured or diseased, the body cannot operate properly. If the problem becomes severe enough, the person involved will consult a physician. The physician will attempt to determine what is causing the problem (make a **diagnosis**), select a treatment, and work with the person, who is now a patient, to either cure or alleviate his or her problem.

Several well-known or common orthopedic problems will be discussed briefly here. The purpose of this section is to acquaint you with various terms you may hear or see written on patients' charts. It will also provide some limited information on how these diseases and disorders are treated, how long the problems may last, and how serious they are. Some orthopedic problems clear up quickly with proper treatment. Others are extremely difficult to treat and may never be cured. It may be important to know the seriousness of the disease in order to understand the reactions of a patient, and be able to treat him or her sympathetically.

INJURIES

The skeleton and the muscles are susceptible to strains, breaks, and tears for two reasons: first, they tend to be on the outside the body. Second, they bear the stresses involved in moving the body and holding it together.

Fractures.

The technical term for any kind of broken bone is **fracture**. There are many different ways of breaking a bone, and each one has a technical name. Only some of the most common types will be covered here (see Figure 64).

1. *Simple (or closed) fracture* A fracture in which the broken bone does not penetrate the skin. A simple fracture leaves no wound on the outside of the body.
2. *Compound (or open) fracture* A fracture in which one or more of the broken bones penetrates the skin.
3. *Greenstick fracture* A partial break in a bone that has not yet completely ossified. This almost always occurs in children, when a bone is bent beyond its limits. The bone splinters on one side only, as a green stick does when it is bent.
4. *Comminuted fracture* A fracture in which the bone is crushed and/or broken into several pieces around the injured area.
5. *Incomplete fracture* A fracture that does not penetrate the entire bone.
6. *Spiral fracture* A break that occurs when a bone is twisted. The fracture makes a spiral-shaped pattern in the bone.
7. *Impacted fracture* A fracture in which one piece of bone is driven into the rest of the bone by the force of the injury.
8. *Silver fork fracture* A break in the lower end of the radius. The name comes from the shape of the bone after such an injury.
9. *Depressed skull fracture* A fracture of the skull in which the broken piece is pressed into the skull.
10. *Compression fracture* A fracture in which bone is crushed, which commonly occurs in porous (osteoporotic) bones.
11. *Complete fracture* A fracture in which the bone breaks all the way across.

Although some fractures are obvious, others are more subtle. Symptoms of fractures include pain, swelling, discoloration, deformity, and loss of use of the affected limb. If the broken ends of the bone lie adjacent to a nerve, the patient may complain of numbness, tingling, or even paralysis of the affected part.

When a fracture is suspected, a physician will order x-rays to find out if the bone is broken and exactly where any breaks are located. Even in a compound fracture where the bone is sticking out of the skin, x-rays are important to to determine whether the bone

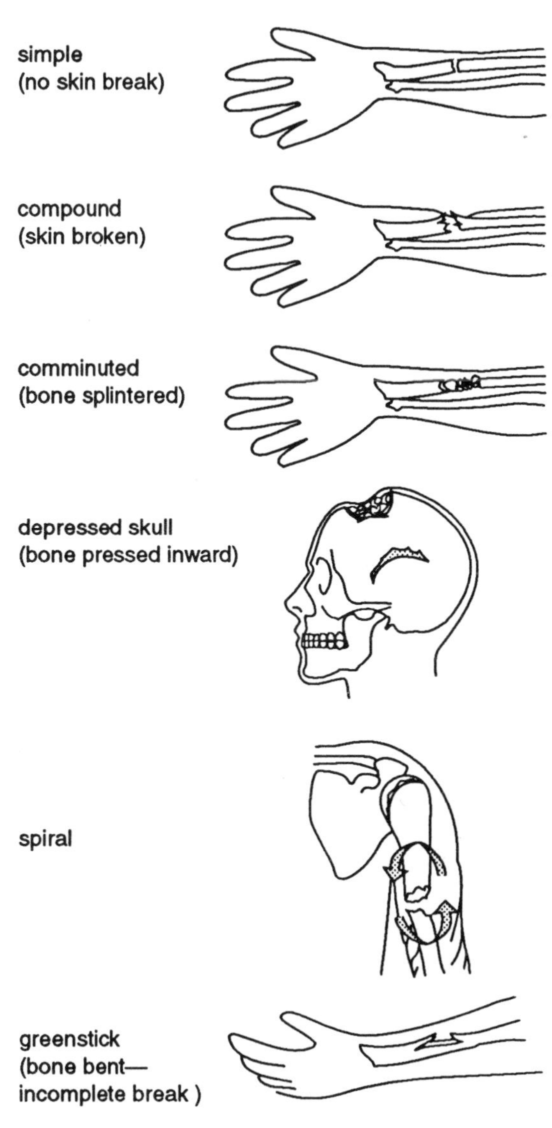

Figure 64: Common fracture types.

is also broken in other places, and also whether fragments of bone are in the wound. X-rays are often used to confirm a diagnosis of bone diseases and injuries. X-rays consist of short wavelength electromagnetic radiation, a classification of energy that also includes radio waves and light. Although x-rays can pass easily through the body, some cell damage may occur. X-ray examinations are generally avoided during pregnancy because of the potential for injuring the fetus.

WARNING!

Young adults suffering fractures of the long bones or pelvis are prone to the development of fat emboli. These emboli may block blood vessels in the brain, kidneys, or lungs, and may occur up to 3 weeks after an injury. Symptoms to be alert for include:

- **sudden increase in temperature, pulse, or respirations**
- **difficulty breathing**
- **mental confusion or coma**

The x-ray machine bombards a photographic film with radiation through the part of the body that is injured. Where the rays reach the film, it becomes dark. The rays can penetrate skin and connective tissue, but not bone, so where the bone intervenes, the film remains white. Any breaks in the bone will show up on the film as shadows, dark spots, or dark lines on the white areas.

An untreated fracture begins to heal almost immediately. The physician has two jobs in treating a fracture. The first is to set the broken bones so that the restored bone is in the right position to heal in the correct shape. The second is to keep the bone there as it heals. Setting the bone in position is called **reduction.** It can be done in two ways. In **closed reduction,** the physician manipulates the bone into place without opening the skin. In **open reduction,** an incision or cut into the site of the fracture is necessary to put the broken bone in place.

Holding the bone in place is called **immobilization.** It can usually be done with a plaster or fiberglass cast or a strong bandage. However, in some cases the bone will not heal properly unless it is put in **traction.** An arrangement of weights or pulleys is set up to put enough tension on the bone and surrounding muscles to hold the bone in place as it begins to heal. To do this, the patient may have to remain in the same position for some time.

WARNING!

X-ray examinations should be used with discretion during pregnancy. Always ask female patients of childbearing age who are scheduled for an x-ray examination whether there is any possibility that they may be pregnant. This will help ensure that adequate radiation shielding is given to the patient's abdominal area during an x-ray study.

An ordinary fracture in an otherwise healthy person usually takes about 4 to 6 weeks to heal completely. In general, the younger the person, the faster it heals. While the bone heals, the muscles around it are not used. They may weaken, or even **atrophy (AT ruh fee)** and special exercises are usually necessary to restore muscle tone.

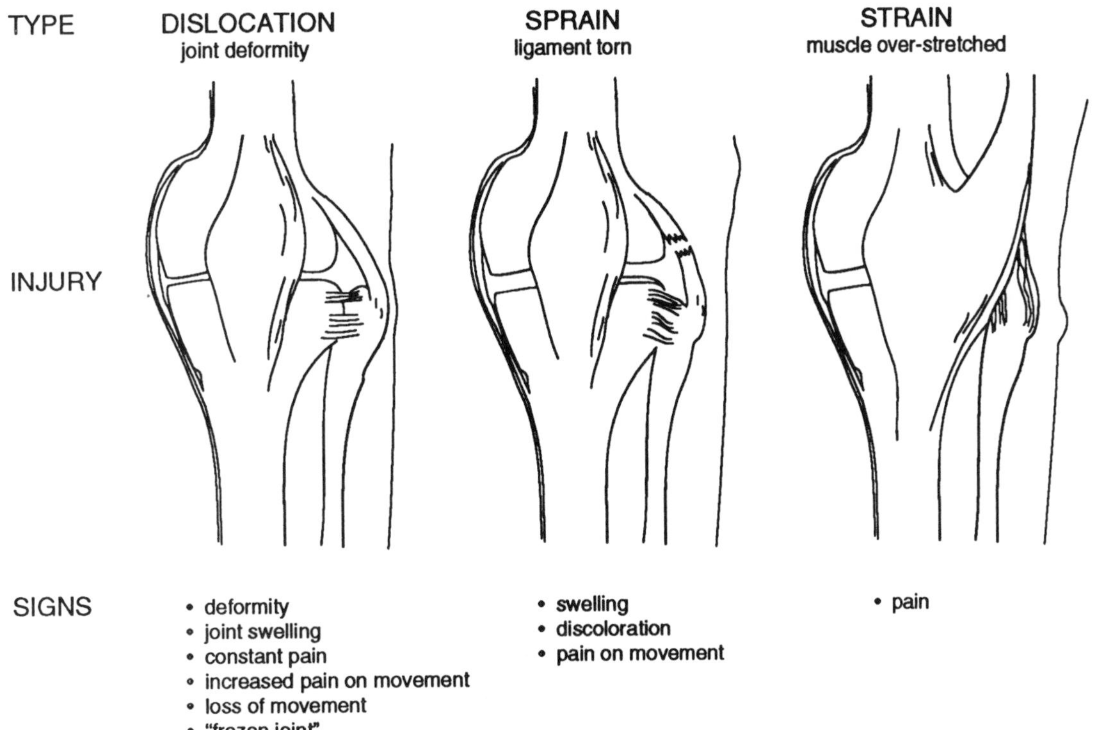

Figure 65: Musculoskeletal injuries other than fractures.

Other Injuries.

Other injuries, or **traumas (TRAW muhs),** that may affect the musculoskeletal system without actually breaking a bone include sprains, strains, dislocations, torn cartilages, severed tendons, and inflammations of tendons or joints.

In a **sprain,** the ligaments around a joint are torn but not severed. A severe sprain causes swelling and pain, and an x-ray may be done to make sure no bones are broken. A sprain is treated by applying heat or cold to reduce swelling, bandaging the joint, and resting the joint and resting until it has a chance to heal by itself. The ligaments usually repair themselves in a week or 10 days.

A **strain** is a torn or overstretched muscle or tendon. Again, the tissue is not severed. A strain is painful and may cause swelling, but the pain is not at the joint (see Figure 65). The term pulled muscle is commonly used to describe a strain. Treatment is rest of the muscle and gradual resumption of movement and use. Strains tend to recur in the same place, especially if the muscle is used too much or too soon before healing is complete.

Dislocation occurs most often in the shoulder or the hip, both of which are ball-and-socket joints. The bones of the joint actually move out of their proper places. They sometimes return to the normal position by themselves, or sometimes they must be put back in place.

The symptoms of dislocation are swelling, deformity, painful movement, and a decreased range of motion of the joint.

It is important to know what you are doing before you try to relocate, or reduce, a dislocated joint. Dislocation involves damage to the ligaments—otherwise the bones would stay in place. The treatment, once the joint is back in place, is to relieve pain and rest the joint. It may have to be bandaged to keep it in place until it heals. If a dislocation recurs several times, surgical repair may be necessary. Sometimes treatment includes putting in a steel pin to hold the bones in place.

Torn cartilage is most common in the knee joint. The cartilage at the ends of the long bones in the thigh or the lower leg is damaged, either by injury or by faulty circulation in the joint area. The symptoms are pain, swelling, and sometimes limited movement of the joint. This condition may heal by itself if the affected joint is rested. However, if the problem persists and worsens, surgery may be necessary. In the operation, the surgeon removes the torn portion of the cartilage and smooths over the end of the bone so that the joint can move without irritation.

A severed tendon is difficult to repair because a tendon is under constant tension. When it is cut, therefore, it snaps back to its origin. Before the injury can heal, the ends of the tendon must be found, stretched back to their normal positions, and stitched together. This may require extensive surgery to locate the ends. An injury that involves a severed tendon may take quite a while to heal because of the disruption caused by the search for the severed ends.

Injury or overuse of a limb can cause inflammation of joints or tendons. Inflammation of a joint is called **bursitis (bur SYE tis),** because the bursa (the sac that holds the joint fluid) is the part of the structure that becomes inflamed. The condition can be caused by a blow to the joint or by irritation from parts of the joint rubbing against each other. Symptoms are pain, swelling, and restricted movement. The treatment is protection of the joint, rest, and sometimes injection of steroid drugs into the joint, or removal of excess fluid from the joint. Bursitis can become chronic if the joint is used again too soon. Surgery may be required to remove the calcium deposits and relieve the inflammation.

Inflammation of the tendon is called **tenosynovitis (TEN oh sye noh VYE tis)** or **tendinitis (TEN din EYE tis).** Tenosynovitis means inflammation of the sheath, or synovium, that encases the tendon. This problem usually is caused by overuse or unaccustomed strain on a tendon. It can also result from a blow, or from an infection of the tendon sheath. Tendinitis is a common cause of pain in the shoulder. In severe cases, the tendon's motion becomes restricted either because the sheath adheres to the tendon, or because the walls of the sheath thicken and reduce the space inside. Treatment of the problem depends on location, cause, and severity. In some cases, it is necessary to enlarge the sheath by cutting it open. In most cases, recovery is complete. (STOP AND REVIEW, page 77.)

DISEASES AND DISORDERS

The muscles, the bones, and the joints, like any other part of the human body, are susceptible to diseases. These diseases can be caused by infection, degeneration, or abnormalities.

Joint Diseases

Several diseases or disorders affect the joints. The terms *rheumatism* and *arthritis* have been used interchangeably for a long time to describe these disorders. Many people do not realize that there are several different kinds of problems that may cause pain in the joints. All are uncomfortable, but some can be treated and cured while others are very difficult to deal with.

Osteoarthritis. The most common of these diseases is **osteoarthritis (OS tee oh ahr THRYE tis),** also called **degenerative joint disease.** Although it can start at almost any age, it is strongly associated with the elderly.

STOP AND REVIEW

1. Match the injury with the description.

a. greenstick fracture		____1.	bone breaks completely across
b. impacted fracture		____2.	no wound shows
c. compound fracture		____3.	one piece of bone is driven into another
d. simple fracture		____4.	bone splinters on one side only
		____5.	broken bones penetrate the skin
		____6.	bone breaks when twisted

2. True/False: X-rays penetrate bone to produce an image on photographic film.
3. True/False: Closed reduction of a fracture is a surgical procedure.
4. True/False: In a strain, a muscle or tendon is torn or overstretched at the joint.
5. True/False: Trauma is another word for injury.

Fill in the blanks for questions 6 through 9.

6. Holding a fractured bone in the correct position while it heals is called________________ ____.
7. Placing a fractured bone in the correct position is called________________ ____.
8. Torn cartilage is most common in the________________ ____joint.
9. The term "pulled muscle" is sometimes used to describe a________________ ____.
10. Circle one: Dislocation occurs most often in
    a. hinge joints
    b. gliding joints
    c. ball-and-socket joints
    d. pivot joints

By the age of 70, 85 percent of the population has some signs of osteoarthritis. The cause of the disease is not known, but apparently in some cases it occurs in a joint that was injured previously.

The disease begins slowly. It softens the cartilage at the joints, causing pain after exercise and stiffness after extended inactivity. In most joints, osteoarthritis is painful but not crippling. The distal finger joints are most commonly affected, followed by the hips, knees, and spine. Osteoarthritis of the major joints can be serious. Radiographic examination may help confirm the diagnosis of osteoarthritis. X-rays of the affected joints show narrowing of the joint space or inappropriate growth of bone into the joint area.

Treatment is aimed at relieving pain and inflammation, usually with aspirin or other anti-inflammatory and pain-relieving drugs. It is also important to rest the affected joints. In severe cases, surgery to replace joints with artificial ones may be necessary. There is no cure for the disease.

Rheumatoid Arthritis. This joint disease is far more severe than osteoarthritis. It usually begins in one or more joints between the ages of 25 and 50, and it eventually spreads to all the active joints in the body. **Rheumatoid arthritis (ROO muh toid ahr THRYE tis)** is much more common in women than in men. Its cause is unknown, but it may be an auto-immune disease.

In rheumatoid arthritis the synovial membranes that surround the joints thicken. This causes inflammation, pain, and stiffness. Nodules or lumps appear beneath the surface of the skin at the joints, and eventually the joints become deformed.

This disease cannot be cured, but its spread can be delayed and the pain can be relieved with medical treatment. At first, the patient may require complete bed rest to recover from the initial attack. Anti-inflammatory drugs, such as aspirin or ibuprofen are prescribed in suitable doses.

Once the initial inflammation has been relieved to some extent, the patient can return to a somewhat active life, but must take frequent rests to relieve pressure on the joints. In some severe cases, gold salts injected into the joints may help relieve pain and inflammation. Heat, appropriate exercise, orthopedic shoes, and walking aids may help the patient remain active for quite some time. Joint replacement may also be necessary.

A form of this disease affects children. It is called **juvenile rheumatoid arthritis**. This form of the disease is accompanied by fever, a rash, and sometimes eye involvement. The treatment is similar to that for the adult disease.

Gout. Still another joint disease, **gout** is considered to be a hereditary form of arthritis. It is caused by deposits of uric acid crystals in affected joints. About 95 percent of all cases of this disease occur in men over age 30. It flares up suddenly, usually during the night, with a crushing, throbbing pain in the big toe. The toe becomes tender, red, and swollen, and remains painful for several days. The attack may be related to an injury, tight shoes, overeating or drinking, or stress, but it may also have no apparent cause. The problem subsides, but it can recur at any time. Later attacks may be closer together, last longer, and involve more joints. Chronic gout may permanently deform joints and may attack and destroy kidney cells. Gout can be diagnosed through examination of aspirated synovial fluid, and by x-rays of affected joints. Gout can be treated and virtually eliminated with medication. The drugs that are prescribed eliminate excess uric aid from the system and dissolve the crystals that have already been deposited in the joints.

Ankylosing Spondylitis. Also called rheumatoid spondylitis or Marie-Strümpell disease, **ankylosing spondylitis (ANK ih loh sing SPON dih LYE tis)** affects the spinal joints. It is a chronic or long-term disease that eventually immobilizes the joints between the vertebrae. It usually affects men, starting between the ages of 20 and 30. The cause is not known.

The first symptoms of ankylosing spondylitis are low back pain and stiffness that is worst in the morning. Pain may also occur in the buttocks, hips, and shoulders. As the joints become frozen (immobilized), the pain stops. Treatment is aimed at keeping the back as flexible as possible for as long as possible. Ample rest, prescribed exercise, and application of heat are important in helping to do this. Pain relievers are also prescribed, but aspirin and steroid drugs are not effective. There is no cure for ankylosing spondylitis. The disease usually lasts 10 to 20 years; then a disease-free period, or remission, occurs. However, the disease may return.

Low Back Pain. Another joint problem that affects the spine is termed **low back pain.** This is one symptom of ankylosing spondylitis, but it is also a symptom of many other joint problems. It is often difficult to tell what is causing low back pain, so it may be treated for some time as a symptom without a definite diagnosis.

Osteoarthritis of the spine is one possible cause of low back pain, and so is rheumatoid arthritis. It could also be the result of muscle strain. In other cases, the cause is a **slipped disk,** also called a *ruptured disk* or *herniated disk.* This condition is sometimes extremely painful. One of the discs of cartilage that serve as cushions between each two vertebrae slips out of place, and two things may happen: First, the vertebrae are no longer protected, and may rub against each other, causing irritation of the surrounding tissues. Second, the disk itself may come in contact with a nerve, which will cause considerable pain. Spinal x-rays, myelography (an x-ray study using a radiopaque contrast medium injected into the subarachnoid space around the spinal cord), computed tomography (CT) scans and magnetic resonance imaging (MRI) scans may be used to locate slipped or herniated discs. Treatment for a slipped disk is pain relievers and complete bed rest for 6 weeks or more. If rest is not effective, surgery may be necessary to remove the disk and/or fuse the involved vertebrae so that they no longer rub against each other. (STOP AND REVEIW, page 80.)

Bone Diseases

The bones as well as the joints can become diseased. Earlier in this text, we have seen how the bone is made and that it is not the simple structure it appears to be. Four major diseases can affect the bone directly.

Osteoporosis. The most common of these major diseases is **osteoporosis (OS tee oh poh ROH sis).** This disorder mainly affects the elderly. As you get older, the bones are weakened because more bone cells are destroyed than are manufactured to replace them. As a result, the bones become weak and brittle and break easily. This process can reach a point where the bones, especially the back bones, are easily crushed by what was once normal stress. Lifting a heavy object can cause a vertebra to be crushed. The symptoms of such a break are low back pain and, eventually, abnormal curvature of the spine.

Osteoporosis occurs gradually. It can be caused by underlying disease that prevents bone renewal, by calcium or vitamin D deficiency, or by lack of physical activity. Treatment usually consists of supplements of vitamin D and calcium, pain-relieving drugs, hormones to promote ossification, and protection of the back. Unless there is a treatable underlying disease, osteoporosis cannot be cured.

Osteomyelitis. Another bone disease is **osteomyelitis (OS tee oh mye eh LYE tis)** an

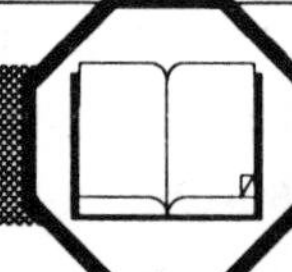

STOP AND REVIEW

Fill in the blanks for questions 1 through 7.

1. Name three causes of diseases or disorders of the muscles and bones.

   a. ____________________

   b. ____________________

   c. ____________________

2. An anti-inflammatory drug that may be prescribed in the treatment of rheumatoid arthritis is ____________________.

3. The joint of the big toe may be affected by deposits of crystals of uric acid in the disease called ____________________.

4. Three causes of low back pain are

   a. ____________________

   b. ____________________

   c. ____________________

5. A disease-free period in the course of a disease is called a ____________________.

6. Describe rheumatoid arthritis, including the part of the joint affected, and the effect the disease has on joint structure. ____________________

   ____

   ____

7. A slipped disk affects the vertebrae above and below it because ____________________

   ____________________.

8. Circle the age group (in years) with which osteoarthritis is most often associated.

   a. 0–10

   b. 11–25

   c. 26–39

   d. 40–69

   e. 70 and over

9. Circle the name of the disease that can be very well controlled with medication.

   a. rheumatoid arthritis

   b. degenerative joint disease

   c. slipped disk

   d. gout

   e. tenosynovitis

10. True/False: Men between the ages of 20 and 30 are those most often affected by rheumatoid arthritis.

infection of the bone marrow. This is caused either by an infection in the body as a whole or by an infectious agent that enters the bone directly from an infected fracture or an infected wound near the bone. The problem is usually caused by *Staphylococcus aureus* bacteria. The symptoms are fever and pain, both of which appear suddenly. The disease may be present for some time before these symptoms occur. If osteomyelitis is not treated, it can destroy the bone cells, leaving a dead and extremely brittle bone in the body. The treatment for osteomyelitis is an antibiotic, usually penicillin, given for an extended period, to cure the infection. The drug is given immediately, and at the same time a culture may be taken from the infection to determine what is causing the problem. If the first drug is not effective, another one more specific to the cause can be prescribed later. However, penicillin will eliminate most causes of the disease. Also, the affected bone must be immobilized, any open infection must be drained, and dead bone must be removed. Osteomyelitis can almost always be cured with antibiotics. The sooner it is discovered and treated, the more effective the treatment will be.

Osteomalacia. A bone disorder caused by a deficiency of calcium and/or vitamin D is called **osteomalacia (OS tee oh muh LAY shee uh).** Both of these elements are necessary for the ossification of bone tissue. Their lack causes the bones to soften. Eventually, the skeleton becomes deformed because the soft bones cannot hold their shape. Osteomalacia sometimes occurs in children and is called *rickets.*

The usual treatment for this problem in adults or children is supplementary doses of the needed nutrients. In some cases the problem occurs because the body cannot absorb these elements, even though they are supplied in the diet. Then treatment is aimed at curing the underlying disorder.

Bone Tumors. The fourth major bone disease is **bone tumors.** Some bone tumors are benign, or noncancerous, but others are malignant, or cancerous. There are many types of bone tumors. Some of the most common benign tumors are called **osteomas (OS tee OH mahs)** and **chondromas (kon DROH mahs).** Some malignant types are **osteosarcoma, (OS tee oh sahr KOH muh)** or osteogenic sarcoma (in the bone), **chondrosarcoma (KON droh sahr KOH muh)** (in the cartilage), and **myeloma (MYE eh LOH muh)** (in the marrow). The main symptom of a bone tumor is pain in the area of growth.

A physician will do a **biopsy (BYE op see)** of a bone tumor to find out what kind it is. In this procedure, a very small section of the tumor is removed and examined under a microscope to see what kind of cells it contains. The treatment for a benign tumor is surgical removal. If the tumor is cancerous, it is removed and either radiation, or drugs **(chemotherapy) (KEE mo THERR uh pee),** or both, are necessary as well. Bone cancer can sometimes be cured, but the rate of cure is generally low. It may be a secondary cancer or **metastasis (meh TAS tah sis),** which means that it has spread from another tumor, often in the lung or the breast. In such cases the disease is usually fatal. (STOP AND REVIEW, page 82.)

Muscle Diseases

Myasthenia Gravis. The muscle tissue is also susceptible to disease. **Myasthenia gravis (MYE as THEE nee uh GRAV is)** is an autoimmune disease that seems to be caused by abnormal transmission of nerve impulses. Because the nerve impulse is faulty, individ-

STOP AND REVIEW

1. Osteoporosis mainly affects what age group? ______________________
2. Deficiency of calcium or vitamin D, or a disease that prevents renewal of bone, can cause ______________________ .
3. A ______________ is performed to find out if a bone tumor is benign or malignant.
4. Place the letter *B* next to benign tumors, and the letter *M* next to malignant ones:
   a. osteoma ______________
   b. osteosarcoma ______________
   c. chondroma ______________
   d. chondrosarcoma ______________
   e. myeloma ______________
5. Circle one: Osteomalacia can be treated with
   a. antibiotics
   b. radiation
   c. dietary supplements
   d. radiation
   e. chemotherapy

ual muscle fibers atrophy or shrink, and this inhibits normal movement. The disease usually starts in the eye and other facial muscles. It may then spread to other parts of the body, and gradually leads to paralysis, or it may go into **remission** and not return for many years. The disease often affects the patient's appearance. The eyelids droop, the smile looks unnatural, and choking on food and speech problems may occur. The patient is often tired, and rest helps the muscles to function better. There are several drugs that give relief.

Muscular Dystrophy (MUS kew lur DIS truh fee). This is another muscle disease that is caused by abnormal muscle function. The disease is inherited, and almost always affects boys. It is not well understood, but it seems to be caused by an inability of the muscle cells to process some substance that they need. The muscles atrophy, but appear large because the atrophied fibers are replaced by connective tissue and fat. The symptoms usually appear between ages 4 and 7, after the child has learned to walk. The child's gait becomes peculiar, and he has trouble standing, because his muscles are weak. The muscles get progressively weaker, so that the child is usually bedridden by his twelfth year and dies by the age of 20 from respiratory problems or heart failure. There is no effective treatment for the disease, but usually the longer the boy remains active the longer he will live.

Tetanus. Two muscle diseases are caused by organisms that enter the body from the outside. **Tetanus (TET ah nus)** is one of these. It is rare in the United States because most people are immunized against it, but it does still occur. Immunization must be renewed at least every least every 5 to 10 years to protect against the disease. The organism that cause tetanus, *Clostridium tetani*, enters the body through a deep wound where air does not penetrate. The organism releases a toxin, or poison, which causes stiffness and eventually rigidity of the muscles. Because stiffness of the jaw is one of the first symptoms of tetanus, this disease is also known as lockjaw.

The disease is painful because of muscle spasms or involuntary contractions. Also, the rigidity of the muscles may make breathing and other body functions difficult. The disease may be of short duration or last for weeks, and recovery is possible if there are no complications. However, complications such as pneumonia are common. Treatment is carried out in an intensive care unit and requires muscle relaxant drugs, help with breathing, complete rest, and careful monitoring to prevent complications.

Trichinosis. The second muscle disease caused by an organism from outside the body is **trichinosis (TRICK ih NOH sis)**. It is due to a parasite that may be found in insufficiently cooked meat, especially pork. There is no way to test meat to see if the organism is present. The only way to prevent this disease is to cook meat thoroughly; the heat of cooking kills the organism.

The disease begins with severe diarrhea as the parasite enters the digestive tract. Then the larvae, or young, of the organism become embedded in the muscle and form calcified cysts, or sacs, in the muscle tissue. This causes weakness, fever, and pain. If the nerves or the heart are involved, the disease can be fatal. Treatment includes extra fluids, adequate diet, and drugs to relieve the pain and fever, and kill the parasite.

Hernia. The final muscle problem we will discuss is the **hernia (HUR nee uh)**. This is not so much a disease as a structural weakness in a muscle. A hernia occurs when an organ, such as the stomach or the intestine, protrudes through the wall that normally contains it. A hernia can be dangerous because the section of organ that is on the "wrong" side of the muscle can become cut off from the rest of the organ and become infected. Severe complications may follow. Also, the function of the organ may be blocked by the hernia.

The least dangerous type of hernia is the **hiatal hernia (hye AY tul)**. In this type, a portion of the stomach protrudes through the diaphragm at the point where the esophagus enters the abdominal cavity. A hiatal hernia rarely causes complications and seldom requires surgery. It does cause heartburn, however. A hiatal hernia can be diagnosed by a gastrointestinal (G.I.) series—an x-ray examination of the upper digestive system. The patient is given barium sulfate (a radiopaque contrast medium) to drink, which outlines the esophagus, stomach, and small intestine on the x-ray films.

Other common types of hernia involve the intestines at various weak points in the abdominal wall. They are the **inguinal (IN gwin al)** hernia, in the groin area; the **umbilical (um BIL ih kal)** hernia, near the navel; the **incisional (in SIH zhun al)** hernia, through the site of an imperfectly healed surgical incision; and the **diaphragmatic (DYE uh frag MAT ick)** hernia, in which the abdominal contents protrude into the thorax through the diaphragm wall. In most cases, these are treated surgically to prevent complications.

Connective Tissue Diseases

Collagen Diseases. There is also a group of diseases that affects the connective tissues. They are called **collagen diseases** because they involve the degeneration of collagen, a gel-like protein that is an essential ingredient of the bones, cartilage, and other connective tissues. These diseases are not well understood, and they are usually fatal, either within a short time or over a period of years, with occasional remissions. Diseases in this category are called **cutaneous lupus erythematosus (kew TAY nee us LOO pus ERR ih the muh TOH sis), systemic lupus erythematosus (SLE), scleroderma (SKLEE roh DUR mah), polymositis (POL ee myel oh SYE tis), dermatomyositis (DUR muh toh MYE oh SYE tis)** and **polyarteritis (POL ee ahr teh RYE tis).** Each one affects different parts of the body, ranging from the skin to the blood vessels. The symptoms vary according to which part is diseased. Treatment is aimed at relieving symptoms, encouraging remissions, and preventing complications.

STOP AND REVIEW

1. Circle the name of the disease that is inherited. Underline the name of the disease that is transmitted in food.
   a. trichinosis
   b. tetanus
   c. muscular dystrophy
   d. osteomalacia
   e. ankylosing spondylitis
   f. myasthenia gravis
   g. chondrosarcoma

Fill in the blanks for questions 2 through 5.

2. Two causes of hernias are____________________ and____________________.
3. Diseases that involve degeneration of the protein____________________ affect the ____________________ tissues, which have ____________________ as an essential ingredient.
4. Osteogenesis imperfecta is a ____________________ bone disorder.
5. The congenital disease achondroplasia affects the formation of cartilage. This means that____.

Congenital Disorders. Finally, there are two disorders, one of the bone and one of cartilage, that are *congenital,* or present at birth. In **osteogenesis imperfecta, (OS tee oh JEN eh sis im pur FECK tuh),** the bones do not develop properly, sometimes starting before birth. As a result of this rare abnormality, the child's skeleton does not form properly, and the bones fracture easily.

Achondroplasia (ah kon dro PLAY zee uh) is the second of these diseases. It affects the formation of cartilage. In this condition also the skeleton cannot form properly, since bone growth takes place in the cartilage. As a result, a child with this congenital problem will grow up with abnormally short bones in the limbs, normal bones in the torso, and abnormal curvature of the spine (lordosis). Achrondroplasia is the most common cause of dwarfism. It accounts for 90 percent of all dwarfs.

Neither of these congenital conditions can be cured. Treatment is designed to make the child's life as life close to normal as possible and, in osteogenesis imperfecta, to try to prevent breakage of bones. Table 19 reviews orthopedic diseases.

Table 19: Review of Orthopedic Diseases

Bone Diseases	Joint Diseases	Muscle Diseases	Connective Tissue Diseases
Bone tumors Benign or malignant abnormal growths	*Osteoarthritis* Degenerative softening of the cartilage, common in elderly	*Myasthenia gravis* Affects transmission of stimuli from nerves, weakens muscle fibers	*Achondroplasia* Congenital defect in cartilage development
Osteoporosis Weakened bone from increased reabsorption of calcium	*Rheumatoid arthritis* Thickened synovium causes deformity; progressive and crippling	*Tetanus* Infection from puncture wound, toxin makes muscles rigid	*Collagen diseases* Collagen in connective tissues degenerates, causing variety of symptoms
Osteomyelitis Infection of bone marrow	*Gout* Uric acid crystals in big toe joint	*Trichinosis* Parasite from meat, larvae in muscle cause weakness	
Osteomalacia Softened bone due to nutritional deficiency	*Ankylosing spondylitis* Spinal joints fuse, become immobilized	*Muscular dystrophy* Affects mainly boys, hereditary, muscles progressively weaken	
Osteogenesis imperfecta Abnormal growth of bone, congenital	*Low back pain* Many causes; may be arthritis, slipped disk, pulled muscle	*Hernia* Weakened muscle wall allows portion of organ to protrude	
	Bursitis Inflammation of bursa		
	Tenosynovitis Inflammation of tendon sheath		

VOCABULARY

A

Abduction *(movement)* Motion of a body part sideways away from the midline.

Acetabulum Socket for hip joint, located where the three parts of the hip bone come together.

Acetycholine Chemical released by a motor neuron that stimulates a muscle.

Achondroplasia Disease that affects formation of cartilage.

Acromion process Ridge on the scapula to which the clavicle is joined.

Actin Protein that is part of a muscle fiber.

Action potential The wave-effect change in electrical charges that follows movement of sodium out of muscle cell.

Adduction *(movement)* Motion of body part toward the midline.

Adductor longus Muscle that moves thigh toward midline.

Adenosine diphosphate Chemical remaining after energy released by a muscle cell after contraction.

Adenosine triphosphate Chemical that provides energy for contraction.

Amphiarthrosis Joint that allows almost no movement, or only a slight amount.

Ankylosing spondylitis Joint disease affecting vertebrae.

Antagonist Muscle that relaxes as the prime mover contracts.

Anterior *(location)* Located toward the front.

Anterolateral *(location)* Located toward the front and side.

Appendicular skeleton The bones of the shoulders, arms, hips, and legs.

Articular cartilage Cartilage covering joints.

Articular surface Cartilage covering joint surfaces.

Articulation Junction or union between two bones.

Atlas First cervical vertebra that supports the head; allows nodding motion.

Atrophy Wasting away of a muscle from disuse.

Auditory meatus Opening in the skull for the ear.

Axial skeleton Bones along center of body from skull to rib cage.

Axis Vertebra that allows the head to turn from side to side.

B

Ball-and-socket joint Joint where rounded end of one bone fits into socket (depression) of another; hip bone, shoulder bone.

Biceps brachii Muscle in front of upper arm.

Biopsy Removal of a sample of tissue for laboratory examination.

Body Inner projection (process) on vertebrae; filled with marrow.

Bone matrix Basic tissue of bone; nonliving material made up of fluids and collagen.

Brachialis Muscle that helps to flex the elbow.

Buccinator Muscle at the side of the mouth.

Bursa (bursae) Sac of membrane filled with fluid that cushions moving parts of a joint.

Bursitis Inflammation of the bursae.

C

Calcaneus Heel bone.

Calcification See Ossification.

Canaliculus (canaliculi) The smallest passageways (carrying nutrients and waste) in bone; part of the haversian system.

Cancellous bone Spongy bone found at the ends of long bones; where growth takes place.

Capitate One of the four distal carpal bones.

Capitulum Rounded projection at lower end of humerus; part of elbow joint.

Cardiac muscle Striated involuntary muscle; heart muscle.

Carpals Eight short wrist bones.

Cartilage Connective tissue lacking blood vessels or canals; flexible tissue attached to the bones.

Chemotherapy Treatment of malignant tumors with cancer-killing drugs.

Cholinesterase Chemical released by a stimulated muscle cell; cholinesterase stops stimulation.

Chondroma Benign bone tumor.

Chondrosarcoma Malignant tumor in cartilage.

Circumduction *(movement)* Circular motion.

Clavicle Collar bone.

Closed reduction Manipulation of a fractured bone into correct position without making an incision.

Coccyx Tailbone.

Collagen diseases Group of diseases that involve degeneration of the protein collagen in connective tissue.

Comminuted fracture Fracture in which bone is crushed into several pieces.

Compact bone Dense bone, like that found in the shaft of long bones. Contains yellow marrow. Also called *cortex.*

Complete fracture Bone broken completely across.

Compound fracture Also called *open fracture;* one or more of the broken bones penetrates the skin.

Concha (conchae) One of three bones in nasal passage.

Costa (costae) Ribs.

Costal cartilage Cartilage that covers ends of ribs where they attach to breastbone, also called *skeletal cartilage.*

Cortex See Compact bone.

Creatine phosphate Chemical released during breakdown of ATP to provide energy for muscle cell contraction.

Cross-bridge Extensions of the myosin (protein) filaments found in a muscle cell; cross-bridges join these filaments to others made of actin.

Cuboid One of the tarsal (foot) bones.

Cuneiform One of the tarsal (foot) bones

D

Degenerative joint disease Diseases such as osteoarthritis that soften cartilage at joints, causing pain or stiffness.

Deltoid Muscle that abducts the arm.

Depressed skull fracture Fracture in which a piece or pieces of the skull bone are pressed into the brain.

Dermatomyositis Disease affecting connective tissue, involving degeneration of collagen.

Diagnosis Determining what causes disease or other medical problem.

Diaphragm Muscle in lower chest, below lungs and above abdominal cavity.

Diaphragmatic hernia Structural weakness in muscle wall where esophagus enters abdominal cavity, also called *hiatal hernia.*

Diaphysis (diaphyses) Shaft of a long bone.

Diarthrosis (diarthroses) Joint structure that allows movement also called *synovial joint.*

Dislocation Bones of a joint (usually shoulder or hip) that are out of normal position.

Distal *(location)* Located away from the body

E

Elastic cartilage Flexible cartilage.

Endomysium Covering of a single muscle cell.

Epicranius Muscle at top of head that raises eyebrows.

Epimysium Covering of groups of muscle cells.

Epiphysis (epiphyses) Area of cancellous bone at ends of long bone, where growth happens.

Ethmoid bone Bone behind nasal bones and in front of sphenoid.

Eversion *(movement)* Turning sole outward.

Extension *(movement)* Opposite of flexion—returning to the anatomical position.

Extensor carpi radialis longus Muscle that extends and abducts hand.

Extensor carpi ulnaris Extends and adducts hand.

Extensor digitorum Muscle that moves fingers.

External intercostal Muscle between ribs that enlarges the chest for inhalation.

External oblique Muscle at side of abdominal cavity.

F

Femur Thigh bone.

Fibrocartilage Somewhat rigid cartilage that joins skeletal bones.

Fibrous cartilage See Fibrocartilage.

Fibula Calf bone.

Flexion *(movement)* Bending movement forward from rest position.

Flexor carpi radialis Muscle that flexes forearm and hand.

Flexor carpi ulnaris Muscle that flexes and adducts hand.

Flexor (Digitorum, profundus, superficialis) muscles that move fingers.

Fontanel Incomplete cranial sutures in infants.

Foramen (foramena) Opening.

Foramen magnum Opening in bottom of occipital bone where spinal column attaches to skull.

Fracture Broken bone.

Frontal *(location)* Located at the front.

Frontalis Front part of epicranus muscle, on forehead.

Frozen Immobilized, as a joint in ankylosing spondylitis.

G

Gastrocnemius Muscle at back of calf.

Glenoid fossa Projection on scapula at shoulder joint.

Gluteus maximus Muscle in buttock.

Glycogen Carbohydrate stored in muscle cells; source of energy for contractions.

Gout Joint disease caused by deposits of uric acid crystals.

Greater multangular One of the four distal carpal bones.

Greenstick fracture Partial fracture of bone that is not completely ossified.

H

Hamate One of the four distal carpal bones.

Hamstring Muscle that flexes lower leg and extends thigh.

Haversian systems Structural units of compact bone that supply nutrients to and remove wastes from bone cells (osteocytes).

Hemopoiesis The process of making blood cells.

Hernia Weakness in muscle wall that allows part of an organ to protrude

Herniated disc Disk of cartilage between two vertebrae that slips out of place.

Hiatal hernia See Diaphragmatic hernia.

Hinge Joint that allows only flexion and extension—as in the elbow.

Humerus Bone of upper arm.

Hyaline cartilage Type of cartilage found in fetus, from which bone develops; also found on ends of bones (articular cartilage) and ribs (costal cartilage).

Hyperextension *(movement)* Bending backward.

I

Iliac crest Curved edge of hip bone.

Ilium Upper portion of pelvic bone.

Ischium Lower portion of pelvic bone.

Immobilization Holding fractured bone in place.

Impacted fracture Piece of fractured bone driven into rest of bone by force of the injury.

Incisional hernia Muscle weakness, caused by imperfectly healed surgical incision, that allows protrusion of an organ through the muscle wall.

Incomplete fracture Fracture in which bone is not broken completely across.

Inguinal hernia Weakness in muscle wall in groin area.

Intercostal Between the ribs; also (external and internal) muscles that enlarge or contract chest during respiration.

Internal oblique Abdominal muscle at side of abdominal cavity.

Inversion *(movement)* Turning sole inward.

Involuntary muscle Muscle not consciously controlled.

Ischium Lowest part of pelvic girdle.

Isometric Muscle contraction in which tension increases while muscle length stays the same.

Isotonic Muscle contraction in which length of fibers shortens while tension remains the same.

J

Joint capsule Extension of periosteum of bones in a joint, which is lined with synovial membrane, filled with synovial fluid, and contains bursae to serve as cushions for moving parts of the joint.

Juvenile rheumatoid arthritis Joint disease affecting children, in which synovial membranes surrounding the joints thicken, causing inflammation, pain and stiffness.

K

Kyphosis Hunchback; condition in which the thoracic region of the spine curves too far outward.

L

Lacrimal bone Bone inside eye socket, along the side of the nose.

Lactic acid By-product of the breakdown of glycogen that supplies energy for muscle contraction.

Lacuna (lacunae) Fluid-filled cavities in bone that surround bone cells. In these cavities the transfer of nutrients and wastes takes place.

Lamella (lamellae) Thin flat sheets of bone matrix surrounding the haversian canals.

Lateral condyle Rounded bulge at knee end of femur that articulates with a similar condyle on the tibia.

Latissimus dorsi Lower back muscle that helps to move the upper arm as well as helping to hold in organs of abdominal cavity.

Lesser multangular One of the four distal carpal bones.

Levator palpebrae superior Muscle that opens eye.

Ligament Strong dense fibrous cords that hold bones together in joint capsules.

Longitudinal arch Arch that runs from heel to toe.

Low back pain Symptom of ankylosing spondylitis or of many other joint problems affecting the spine.

Lunate One of the four proximal carpal bones.

M

Malleolus A process (projection) of the fibula (lateral malleolus) or the tibia (medial malleolus).

Mandible Lower jaw bone.

Masseter Muscle that lifts the lower jaw (mandible).

Maxilla (maxillae) Upper jaw bone.

Medial *(location)* Located at the midpoint.

Medial condyle Rounded bulge at knee end of tibia; articulates with lateral condyle of femur.

Medial epicondyle (funny bone) Projection on the side of the humerus.

Medullary cavity Central cavity in bone that contains marrow.

Metacarpal One of five hand bones.

Metatarsal One of five foot bones.

Metastasis A second cancer that spreads from the site of the original cancer.

Motor neuron Nerve that provides electrical impulse that stimulates muscles to contract.

Muscle fiber Individual muscle cell.

Muscular dystrophy Hereditary muscle disease, usually affecting boys, apparently caused by inability of muscle cells to process some needed substance.

Myasthenia gravis Disease caused by abnormal transmission of nerve impulses that causes muscles to atrophy.

Myeloma Malignant tumor of the bone marrow.

Myofibril Bundles of tiny filaments that are part of a muscle cell.

Myosin A protein found in myofibrils.

N

Navicular One of the seven tarsal or carpal bones.

Normal lordosis Slight inward curve of cervical and lumbar regions of the spine.

Nucleus (nuclei) Central part of cell.

O

Oblique (superior and inferior) Muscles at center of eye socket; (external and internal) outer and inner muscles at sides of abdomen.

Occipital Bone at bottom rear of skull.

Occipitalis Rear part of epicranius muscle found at top of head.

Odontoid process Projection on the axis (second cervical vertebra) that serves as a pivot for the head.

Olecranon Hook-shaped projection at the top of the ulna that fits humerus at the elbow joint.

Open fracture Compound fracture; a fracture in which one or more of the broken bones penetrates the skin.

Open reduction Incision made into site of a fracture so that broken bones can be put back in place.

Orbicularis oculi Muscle around the eye socket that closes eye.

Orbicularis oris Muscle around mouth that purses lips.

Orthopedics Branch of medicine concerned with treating the musculoskeletal system.

Ossification Process of hardening of bones by depositing of calcium and other minerals.

Osteoarthritis Degenerative joint disease, associated with aging, that softens cartilage at the joint, causing pain after exercise and stiffness after inactivity.

Osteoblast Bone-forming cell.

Osteoclast Bone-destroying cell.

Osteocyte Living bone cell.

Osteogenesis imperfecta Congenial disorder in which the bones do not form properly.

Osteogenic sarcoma See Osteosarcoma.

Osteomalacia (rickets) Bone disorder (softening of bone) caused by deficiency of calcium and/or vitamin D.

Osteoma Benign bone tumor.

Osteomyelitis Infection of the bone marrow, usually caused by *Staphylococcus aureus.*

Osteoporosis Condition in which more bone cells are destroyed than are manufactured.

Osteosarcoma Malignant bone tumor.

Oxidative phosphorylation Process that combines ADP, creatine phosphate, and oxygen to recreate ATP (the usual fuel for muscle contraction).

Oxygen debt Condition created when muscle gets energy from glycogen rather than ATP.

P

Palatine bone Bone in roof of mouth.

Palmaris longus Muscle attached to humerus that flexes the hand.

Parasite Organism living within another organism that harms the host organism.

Parathormone Hormone made by parathyroid glands that stimulates the breaking down of bone tissue.

Parietal Bones forming most of the roof and sides of the cranium.

Patella Knee cap; only named sesamoid bone in the body.

Pectoralis major Muscle at front of chest that adducts and rotates arm.

Pelvic girdle Two pelvic bones that support the legs and protect some internal organs.

Perimysium Covering of group of muscle cells.

Periosteum Outer covering of bone.

Phalanx (Phalanges) One of fourteen finger bones.

Pisiform One of four proximal carpal bones.

Pivot Joint that allows rotation.

Platysma Muscle at front of neck that pulls down lower jaw and lower lip.

Polyarteritis See Collagen diseases.

Polymyositis Polymuositis See Collagen diseases.

Posterior *(location)* At the back.

Posterolateral *(location)* Side back.

Prime mover Muscle that exerts a major pulling force.

Process Projection on a bone.

Pronation *(movement)* Turning palms downward or backward.

Protraction *(movement)* Lowering jaw/sticking out tongue.

Proximal *(location)* Nearest to body.

Pterygoid Four muscles that move lower jaw side to side for chewing or speech.

Pubis Front part of pelvic bone.

Q

Quadriceps femoris Four-part muscle at front of thigh that flexes thigh and extends lower leg.

R

Radius (radii) Smaller of the two forearm bones.

Rectus abdominis Extension of abdominal oblique muscles, located in front of the abdominal cavity.

Red marrow Marrow made up of connective tissue, blood vessels, and cells that make red and white blood cells.

Reduction Placement of fractured bones back in correct position for healing.

Remission Disease-free period in the course of a disease.

Retraction *(movement)* Raising jaw or pulling back tongue.

Rheumatoid arthritis Joint disease in which synovial membranes surrounding the joints thicken, causing inflammation, pain, and stiffness.

Rickets (osteomalacia) Softening and deformity of bones caused by deficiency of calcium and/or vitamin D.

Rotation *(movement)* Pivoting motion.

S

Sacroliac joint Joint where ilium (upper portion of pelvic bone) articulates with sacrum (vertebra at base of spine).

Sacrum Vertebra at base of spine.

Saddle joint Joint (such as thumb at wrist) allowing five kinds of movement.

Sarcolemma Outer membrane of muscle cell.

Sarcomere Unit of a myofibril; unit of contraction.

Sarcoplasm Main body of muscle cell.

Sarcoplasmic reticulum Network of canals with sacs containing calcium at the ends of them; found in sarcoplasm.

Sartorius Muscle at front of hip that flexes and adducts the lower leg.

Scapula (scapulae) Shoulder blade.

Scleroderma See Collagen diseases.

Scoliosis Abnormal vertical curvature of the spine.

Secondary cancer Cancer that has spread from another tumor located elsewhere in the body.

Sella turcica Depression on upper surface of the sphenoid bone in the skull it holds the pituitary gland.

Semispinalis capitis Muscle at back of neck that moves the head back and sideways.

Sesamoid bone Small bones (mostly unnamed) found in joints.

Shoulder girdle The two clavicles and two scapulae that attach the arms to the axial skeleton.

Silver fork fracture Break in lower end of radius.

Simple fracture Fracture in which broken bones do not penetrate skin.

Sinus Cavity in facial or cranial bones; parts of the respiratory system.

Skeletal cartilage Another name for articular and costal cartilage together.

Slipped disk (herniated disk) Condition in which one of the intervertebral discs that cushion the vertebrae is out of position.

Soleus Muscle in the back of the lower leg that, with the gastrocnemius, forms the calf.

Sphenoid bone Bone that holds all cranial bones except the temporal bones in place.

Spiral fracture Break occurring when bone is twisted; fracture makes a spiral-shaped pattern.

Sprain Injury in which ligaments around a joint are torn but not severed.

Sternocleidomastoid Muscles at front of neck that pull head forward and sideways.

Strain Torn or overstretched (but not severed) muscle; not located at joint.

Striated muscle Muscle that, under the microscope, appears to have striations or bands in it.

Summation Double contraction stimulus of a muscle.

Supination *(movement)* Turning palms upward or forward.

Suture Union between bones, filled with cartilage and fibrous connective tissue, that allows little or no movement.

Synarthrosis Union in which bones are held rigidly together.

Synergist Muscle that acts with a prime mover, to help the movement or to hold the moving part stable.

Synovial fluid Fluid inside a joint capsule.

Synovial joint Diarthrosis; joint that allows movement.

Synovial membrane Slippery, moist lining of joint capsule.

T

T-tubules Dividers in sarcomeres that form the Z-line; part of the mechanism of contraction.

Talus One of seven tarsal bones that forms a joint with the lower leg bones.

Tarsal Seven bones between lower leg and metatarsals (foot bones).

Temporal Bones at lower part of side of head, in which there are openings for the ears.

Tendonitis Inflammation of the tendon.

Tendon Strong, dense fibrous cords that attach muscles to bones.

Tenosynovitis Inflammation of the covering of the tendon.

Tetanus Muscle contraction resulting from stimuli that continue in rapid succession. Also, disease caused by *Clostridium tetani.*

Tibia Shinbone.

Tibialis anterior Muscle at front of lower leg that flexes the foot.

Torn cartilage Damage to cartilage at the ends of bones.

Traction Method of immobilization that also puts tension on bone and surrounding muscles to hold it in place while healing.

Transverse abdominis Inner layer of muscle on the sides of the abdomen.

Transverse arch Arch running from side to side of foot.

Transverse tubule See T-tubule.

Trapezius Muscle covering scapula; works with the other shoulder muscles; alone, it draws the scapula up and toward the spine.

Trauma Injury.

Triangular One of the four proximal carpal bones.

Triceps brachii Muscle at back of upper arm that extends the arm.

Trichinosis Muscle disease caused by parasites found in uncooked meat or meat not thoroughly cooked.

Trochlea Rounded projection on the lower end of the humerus that forms part of the elbow joint.

Trochanter (greater and lesser) Bulges in top of femur, just below its head.

Troponin Chemical that inhibits contraction of muscle cells.

Twitch Single jerky contraction of a muscle in response to a single unrepeated stimulation.

U

Ulna Longest bone in forearm.

Umbilical hernia Weakness in muscle wall near navel that allows abdominal organs to protrude

V

Visceral muscle Smooth involuntary muscle.

Volkmann's canals Openings through which microscopic veins and arteries penetrate bone.

Voluntary muscle Striated (skeletal) muscle that is consciously controlled.

Vomer Bone at base and rear of nasal passage.

Y

Yellow marrow Marrow containing connective tissue blood vessels, fat cells, and cells that make white blood cells.

Z

Z-line Boundary line formed by T-tubules within myofibrils that are part of the mechanism of contraction.

Zygomatic bone Cheek bone.

INDEX